The Cleveland Clinic Guide to

HEART FAILURE

The Cleveland Clinic Guide to

HEART
FAILURE

Randall C. Starling, MD, MPH

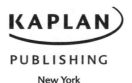

PUBLISHING

New York

This publication is designed to provide accurate and authoritative information in regard to the subject matter covered. It is sold with the understanding that the publisher is not engaged in rendering medical, legal, or other professional service. If medical advice or other expert assistance is required, the services of a competent professional should be sought.

Heart cross section, page 17: Reprinted with the permission of The Cleveland Clinic Center for Medical Art & Photography © 2009.

Published by Kaplan Publishing, a division of Kaplan, Inc.
1 Liberty Plaza, 24th Floor
New York, NY 10006

Printed in the United States of America

10 9 8 7 6 5 4 3 2 1

Library of Congress Cataloging-in-Publication Data
Starling, Randall C., 1951-
The Cleveland Clinic guide to heart failure/Randall C. Starling.
    p. cm.
  Includes index.
  ISBN 978-1-60714-074-0
  1. Heart failure—Popular works. I. Cleveland Clinic Foundation.
II. Title.
  RC685.C53S729 2009
  616.1'29–dc22
                                                2009007255

Kaplan Publishing books are available at special quantity discounts to use for sales promotions, employee premiums, or educational purposes. Please email our Special Sales Department to order or for more information at *kaplanpublishing@kaplan.com*, or write to Kaplan Publishing, 1 Liberty Plaza, 24th Floor, New York, NY 10006.

Contents

Preface

Taking the "failure" out of heart failure—an open letter to new heart failure patients from an old hand

So, you have just been told you have heart failure. My guess is that it is a little overwhelming to learn that you have joined a club that over the years has become increasingly less exclusive.

In the course of the next few months, you will be provided with all sorts of information about how your heart functions, new medications and their purpose, changes in diet, and the cessation of one or two unhealthy indiscretions. It is a lot to take in, and you may not be in the mood right now.

Even the name of the condition isn't particularly conducive to helping you cope. You have to wonder which bright spark decided to call it "heart failure." The word *failure* really isn't a good place to start is it? So how about we call it HF and pretend the *F* stands for something else. (Polite suggestions only please.)

As an alternative to the masses of booklets being given to you, I thought you might like to hear from someone who has been through the adventure you are just starting. And trust me, it is an adventure. Like any adventure, it has ups and downs. But that's how life is anyway, right?

First, a little about me; in addition to her sense of humor, my mother decided to pass to me the cardiac condition that she inherited from her mother. I got my first pacemaker when I was 19 years old. The most recent device, the seventh, is a defibrillator, for which I have been immensely grateful on more than one occasion. I developed HF in 2003.

It is easy to feel swamped by your new circumstances, but it needn't be that way so long as you can develop positive coping mechanisms. This may sound easier than it is, but there are plenty of people that want to assist you. In order to help, here are some pearls of wisdom.

At the outset, it is important to know there is no right or wrong way to cope. There is only one way, your way. Yes, it will take an effort, and yes, at times it is possible to become a little obsessive as you try to stick to your new boundaries. However getting motivated is key.

My own approach has been to intellectualize HF. I have always been interested in complex problems, and HF is the mother of complex problems. (Fortunately my doctors aren't so fazed.) I have to admit at times I even find my situation fun. Peculiar, huh? I am sure you will find your own way to be motivated and maintain a positive outlook.

It is likely that over the years to come, you will spend more time visiting hospitals than you would like. It is best to do everything you can to limit those days to outpatient appointments. Let's face it, who wants to put up with the taste-free food so thoughtfully provided by the hospital when you are admitted as an inpatient? (I seem to have been particularly cursed by low-sodium tomato soup.)

The best way to avoid an emergency admission is to remember that two main reasons lead to HF patients checking in. Not carefully following their medication regime is one. The other is throwing caution to the wind and ignoring the dictary advice. The latter can be particularly challenging if you happen to see someone munching on a delicious-looking pizza. However, it really is possible to cook tasty food without salt. New food is just part of the adventure.

Life will become easier if you engage with your doctor effectively. Over the years, I have been cared for by some truly wonderful health care professionals, all of whom have made it clear they are here to help. To get the most out of them, it essential to join them in partnership with your own health care. They can't work alone; you have to be in the game, too.

Some people worry about asking questions of their doctors, fearing that they may offend or perhaps simply not understand the answers. The fact is that doctors like to be asked questions, as doing so demonstrates you are working with them. The concepts and jargon can be complicated and difficult to understand. Don't worry; there is no answer too confusing that it cannot be distilled down to simple, comprehensible analogies.

If you don't understand what you are being told, say so and ask for a simpler explanation. One good way to check your understanding is to say what you think you have heard; your doctor will quickly set you straight if you have misunderstood.

As we all know, doctors are busy bunnies, and it is not always possible to keep them pinned down until you have had your questions comprehensively answered. Or perhaps something will pop into your mind some hours later. Fear not, there are endless sources of help. It may take a little time, but your questions will be answered.

A word of caution; there is plenty of useful information on the Internet. There is also, frankly, plenty out there that should have a health warning. Just because a Web site says something doesn't mean it applies to you or you should worry about it. Remember that "having information is not the same as understanding it."

With all the information coming in your direction, you will need to take time to reflect on what you have been told. Many in the health care industry believe that a significant proportion of patients don't have the intellectually capacity to understand their medical issues. My response is "hogwash!" If you can understand how to buy and use a cell phone, then you can understand the basics of your condition. It really isn't that hard. Try not to stew over things you don't understand. With a little application, you will understand.

It is essential to recognize that the human body is a finely balanced organism. Even doctors don't fully understand how everything works together. Sometimes it is difficult to see how some symptoms are related to HF, but they are, though you may have difficulty making the connection.

Think of it this way: Have you ever driven down the highway and suddenly found the traffic grinding to a slow crawl? When you get to the cause, sometimes it is an accident on the other side of the barrier. You may wonder how an accident in the opposing traffic can cause a scrunch on your side of the road. The two should be completely unrelated, but they clearly aren't. When one bit of the road network has problems, it always creates disturbances elsewhere.

The human body is the same. Subtle interactions are not obvious at first when you think about HF. Heart pumping efficiency, hormonal activity, chemical imbalances, fluid accumulation, and even electrical short-circuits are part and parcel of the HF game. Your body, your diet, and your medications are all trying to reach some sort of equilibrium. It may take a little time to get to a comfortable steady state, and doing so will certainly require a little experimentation. There is no magic wand to fix HF; your body is far too delicate and intricate for that.

Now for a brief word about your family. Often it is easier for the patient to deal with HF than for relatives. You are actually living with HF. Your family, on the other hand, are standing outside your bubble and observing, without having any real control or a thorough understanding of what you are dealing with. This lack of control can be frustrating to them and the cause of anxiety, which may have an effect on you. If you show them you are confident and feel, to some degree, in control, your poise can make life a little bit easier for everyone. Personally, I am very happy to have my hospital appointments on my own; I have been a heart patient for 36 years and know the routine. You on the other hand, might want to have a whole posse with you for comfort. Sharing the burden is generally good for everyone involved.

Finally, the most important thing to remember is to try to stay positive. At times this can be darn difficult, but I have learned that I always come out from the dark into the sunshine. With the right attitude, so will you. I certainly wouldn't choose to have HF, but now that I have it, I will make the most of it. As a result of my condition, I have met lots of new people, made some wonderfully close friends, and been on the receiving end of mind-boggling kindness and generosity. It may sound weird, but at times this adventure has been hilariously funny. All things considered, I consider myself very lucky.

For me, this is just another test that life has put in my path, albeit a significant one. I am determined not to let it defeat me, and hopefully you won't let if defeat you either.

Stephen Bacon
Cambridge, United Kingdom

Introduction

When I met Dan in 2004, it was hard to picture the active outdoorsman he once was. At 44 years old, he had suffered from Becker's muscular dystrophy for more than a decade. The inherited disorder slowly weakened the muscles in his legs, buttocks, hands, and eventually his heart.

Dan underwent a series of treatments for heart failure at Cleveland Clinic. Doctors here implanted a pacemaker, then a left ventricular assist device to manage Dan's condition while he waited for a donor heart. In June 2005, Dan received a heart transplant. It gave him a new lease on life, allowing him to hike and hunt once again in the forests of the Appalachian Mountains he so loves.

Dan's story is one of hope, and his is not the only one. When patients discover that they have heart failure, they're typically filled with dread. Let's face it: any diagnosis containing the word *failure* doesn't sound promising. But with recent advancements in medicine, people have good reason to remain optimistic that even with heart failure, they can survive and enjoy a good quality of life.

Fifteen to 20 years ago, we more or less treated everybody the same way: with two or three pills. That was all we had to offer. The clock continued ticking while we waited until patients were so sick that they needed heart transplants. The medical landscape is completely different today.

Now we methodically dissect cases of heart failure and figure out the underlying issues. Although heart failure is the diagnosis, it's also an indicator that something else is wrong. So we check for abnormal heart rhythms, problems with electrical conduction, primary muscle problems, blocked arteries, valve troubles, and more.

It's critical to have a timely and proper diagnosis, but it's equally important to determine the cause of the heart failure, which, in turn dictates the best way for it to be treated. Once we figure out the root problem, we have lots of very effective treatments, ranging from medication, to cardiac devices, to surgical procedures.

In many cases, we can essentially reverse the symptoms and return debilitated patients to their previously active lifestyles. Perhaps even more exciting, we can change the structure of their hearts from enlarged and weak to smaller and stronger with the therapies we have to offer today. With proper care, people with heart failure can continue enjoying life and their favorite activities.

That's great news and reason to read on. This book discusses the causes of heart failure and how it's treated.

It provides advice for those living with heart failure and highlights cutting-edge research that is further advancing the field. It's not meant to be a comprehensive textbook but rather a basic guide and beacon of hope.

Not all stories about patients with heart failure have happy endings, but many do. Throughout this book, you'll find stories about patients just like Dan, who triumphed over their diagnosis. Whether it's you, a family member, or a friend confronting heart failure, we hope that this book helps steer you through the diagnosis and treatment, come to terms with your new circumstances, and get on with your life.

Randall C. Starling, MD, MPH
Professor of Medicine
Section Head, Heart Failure and Cardiac
Transplant Medicine
Medical Director, Kaufman Center for Heart Failure
Vice Chairman, Cardiovascular Medicine
Cleveland Clinic

PART I

What You Need to Know About Heart Failure

Chapter 1

What Is Heart Failure?

B efore we delve into details about heart failure, it's important to have a basic understanding of how a healthy heart functions. Your heart is a muscle that acts as a pump, beating approximately 100,000 times a day. It's only about the size of your fist, but it's responsible for feeding the rest of your body's organs oxygen-rich blood.

The heart's robust, muscular walls contract and expand in synchrony, pushing five or six quarts of blood throughout your body each minute. Your brain, kidney, liver, lungs, stomach, and other vital organs require oxygen-rich blood in order to properly perform their respective functions. A healthy heart ensures proper circulation and provides oxygen-rich blood to these organs.

Your heart is divided into two sides, which work in tandem and are separated by an inner wall called the *septum.* The right side pumps blood to your lungs to pick up oxygen. Next the oxygenated blood returns from the lungs to the left side of the heart, which pumps it to the rest of your body.

Your heart has four chambers—two on each side—and four sets of valves. The upper chambers (the right and left *atriums*) receive blood from *veins,* while the lower ones (the right and left *ventricles*) pump blood into *arteries.* Blood enters the right atrium through two large veins and flows to the right ventricle through the open *tricuspid valve.* It leaves the heart through the *pulmonary valve,* travels through the *pulmonary artery,* and then enters the lungs.

Oxygenated blood returns from the lungs to the left atrium and moves through the open *mitral valve* into the left ventricle. The left ventricle pumps blood out of the heart, through the *aortic valve,* and into the *aorta* from where the blood travels on its way around the body in a network of arteries.

The heart is a finely tuned machine: it must contract with enough strength to circulate blood throughout the body, yet it also needs to relax between beats so that it can fill adequately with blood. If any part of this elaborate system breaks down, heart failure may occur.

Mike

It was April 4, 2005, Opening Day for Major League Base-ball. Mike and his wife, Michelle, headed down to the winding banks of the Ohio River to watch the Cincinnati Reds take on the New York Mets. This was an annual tradition for the couple, who had gone to an Opening Day Reds game on their first date. Now they had been married for a dozen years.

Mike and Michelle witnessed an exciting game, with their home team rallying from behind in the ninth inning to beat the Mets 7–6. While Mike was happy that the Reds had won, he wasn't in the mood for any postgame celebration. "We went down for the two o'clock game, and I kept saying to my wife, 'I don't feel so well,'" he recalls. "I got out of breath quickly. I just felt blah."

A few days later, Mike was convinced that he had the flu: he was bone tired and suffering from nausea and diarrhea. As a busy real estate agent representing a new-home building con-tractor, Mike didn't have time to be sick. "I thought, 'Let's see if I can sweat this out of my system.' So I exercised. That didn't work, I actually collapsed in my garage one afternoon and didn't tell my wife for two days. I just kept on going."

In addition to his being unable to keep down food, Mike's upper back hurt; it felt as if he had pulled a muscle. For two weeks, Mike endured the flulike symptoms, pulling himself out of bed and slogging through the day, only to end up back in bed before nightfall. Then on April 18, he coughed up blood. "My wife said, 'That's it! You're going to the doctor,'" he says.

The family physician listened to Mike's lungs and heard rattling. He ordered a chest X-ray. When the results from the radiologist arrived the next day, the doctor told Mike, "It looks like you bought yourself a three-day stay in the hospital. You have influenza and pneumonia, and you need antibiotics."

Admitted to a Mercy Health Partners hospital in Cincinnati, Mike learned that he had more serious medical problems. Looking at the X-ray used to diagnose the pneumonia, doctors discovered that the lower part of Mike's heart was swollen. Mike was sent across town to the Christ Hospital and underwent an echocardiogram and an angiogram. "Until that point, I still thought I just had the flu," he says.

But two weeks later, at age 42, Mike felt his world turn upside down when he was told that he had heart failure. He wasn't alone: approximately 550,000 people are diagnosed with the condition each year. (The rest of Mike's story appears in chapter 6.)

A Basic Explanation of Heart Failure

Heart failure is a misleading term. The heart does not stop functioning, as the word *failure* suggests. And a diagnosis of heart failure does not indicate that the heart is about to stop working. Instead heart failure simply means that the heart's pumping power is diminished and can't circulate enough blood throughout the body.

Heart failure is a *syndrome*, or group of symptoms that collectively characterize the disease. It occurs when the heart muscle is damaged or overworked, typically as a result of other diseases or conditions. It rarely comes on out of the blue but develops over time as the pumping action of the heart progressively weakens. Heart failure is usually a chronic condition, and it can affect the left side, right side, or both sides of the heart.

With heart failure, blood travels throughout the body more slowly, and as a result, pressure in the heart increases. The heart is no longer able to pump sufficient oxygen and nutrients to feed the body. Its four chambers respond either by stretching to hold more blood or by thickening or stiffening. These compensatory responses help keep blood moving for a short time, but as the cardiac muscles weaken, the heart simply can't pump forcefully enough. As a result, patients like Mike feel weak and out of breath.

Are there different types of heart failure?

Rarely in the medical community are conditions so straightforward that they're given one name only. That's true of heart failure too. You may hear your physician talk about congestive heart failure or diastolic heart failure. In all, there are five terms you may encounter, which I've described below.

Left-sided heart failure. Also called *left ventricular heart failure,* this involves one of the heart's lower chambers. While heart failure can affect the left, right, or both sides of the heart, it typically compromises the left side first, as in Mike's case.

Oxygen-rich blood moves from the lungs to the left atrium, then to the left ventricle, which pumps it to the body. In patients with left-sided heart failure, the heart is unable to pump enough blood either due to *systolic* or *diastolic* failure (explained below). In both cases, blood entering the left ventricle may accumulate, causing fluid to seep into the lungs. In addition, as the heart's pumping action decreases, blood flow slows. This may cause *edema:* a buildup of fluid in tissues throughout the body.

Right-sided heart failure. The right atrium receives blood as it returns to the heart through the veins. The right ventricle then pumps it into the lungs, where the blood picks up oxygen. When heart failure affects the right side of the heart, it becomes unable to pump sufficient blood to the lungs. As a result, the incoming blood backs up in the body's veins, which often causes the ankles and legs to swell.

Congestive heart failure. When the heart muscle fails, the kidneys may respond by retaining water and sodium in the body. As fluid builds up in the arms, legs, feet, lungs, or other organs, the body becomes congested. This condition is called *congestive heart failure.*

Diastolic heart failure. This form gets its name because the problem happens during the *diastole* period of the heart's activity: when the heart relaxes after a beat. The heart muscles stiffen and are unable to fill adequately with blood during the resting period, so the heart lacks sufficient blood to pump out. As the heart chamber thickens, there's little room for the heart to relax, and blood backs up in the lungs. The blood pressure increases in the heart and lungs, causing shortness of breath. At first, this occurs only with exertion, but eventually, in severe cases, it happens when the person is at rest or with minimal activities, such as talking or dressing.

Systolic heart failure. This type of heart failure acquires its name because of problems during the *systole* period of the heart's activity, or when it is pumping blood out to the rest of the body. The left ventricle heart muscle becomes unable to contract with enough vigor, so less oxygen-rich blood is delivered out into the arteries and pumped through the body. *Systolic heart failure* results in a reduced *ejection fraction*. This is the proportion of blood that leaves the heart each time it contracts. A normal ejection fraction is in the range of 55 percent to 65 percent. Patients with systolic heart failure typically have an ejection fraction of less than 50 percent and, in severe cases, as low as 10 percent to 15 percent.

Many patients with heart failure have both systolic and diastolic heart failure. Approximately 40 percent of patients have isolated diastolic heart failure, which is often associated with other illnesses such as hypertension, coronary artery disease, and diabetes.

Who's at risk?

Heart failure seems to be an equal opportunity condition, in that it can happen to anyone. However, according to the National Heart, Lung, and Blood Institute, it is more prevalent in people age 65 or older and in African-Americans.

Although men have a higher rate of heart failure than women, the condition affects more elderly women because they typically live longer.

Consider these overall statistics about heart failure:

- Nearly 5 million Americans are affected by heart failure.
- Heart failure is the single most frequent cause of hospitalization for people 65 or older.
- At age 40, the lifetime risk of developing congestive heart failure for both men and women is 1 in 5, according to a study by the National Heart, Lung, and Blood Institute.

Ironically, medical advancements have led to an increase in the number of people diagnosed with heart failure. People are living longer as a result of surviving heart attacks and other conditions, thus increasing their odds for developing heart failure later in life.

What are the symptoms of heart failure?

When you're diagnosed with heart failure, the condition is likely to affect far more than just your heart. Heart failure is a systemic illness that can impair your breathing, sleeping, eating—any activity essential to daily living. And because heart failure is a syndrome, it may impinge on many other organs.

Unfortunately, there's no simple checklist of symptoms common to all heart failure patients. In most people, the damaged heart produces noticeable symptoms. Occasionally, however, people remain unaware that they have seriously impaired hearts. Someone with heart failure may have one, all, or none of the following symptoms, which may persist or come and go and may be mild or severe.

Shortness of breath. Breathing becomes labored when fluid builds up in the lungs, a condition that physicians refer to as *pulmonary edema* or *congestion.* People with heart failure may experience breathlessness not only during activity or exercise but also while they rest or sleep. Sometimes they have trouble lying flat and need to prop up their heads and upper bodies on pillows. (Doctors call this condition *orthopnea.*) In addition, the shortness of breath may come on suddenly, waking people from a sound sleep. (Physicians have a name for this too: *paroxysmal nocturnal dyspnea,* or *PND.*) It is important to describe these symptoms every time you visit your heart failure specialist for a checkup because they mean that your treatment needs to be adjusted.

Coughing or wheezing. This symptom, too, is caused by fluid backing up in the lungs. People with heart failure often suffer from a persistent dry, hacking cough or a cough that produces white or pink blood-tinged mucus. Your doctor will determine whether your cough is from heart failure, another condition, or perhaps your medication.

Fatigue. When the heart is unable to pump enough blood to feed the body's tissues, the body compensates by redirecting blood from less critical organs, such as muscles in the limbs, and sending it to the heart and brain. This causes people with heart failure to feel very tired most of the time. Everyday tasks, including walking, climbing stairs, and taking a shower, become difficult. When simple tasks cause breathlessness, it's called *dyspnea.*

Swelling. Swelling, also called edema, occurs because less blood travels to the kidneys, resulting in fluid and water retention. People with heart failure may experience swollen ankles, feet, legs, or abdomens. They often complain that their shoes feel too tight.

Dizziness or confusion. Severe heart failure and low cardiac output can alter the levels of certain substances in the blood, such as sodium, which in turn may impair thinking. Family members, friends, or caregivers may be the first to notice someone's poor memory or disorientation. In addition, heart failure may also increase the chance of blood clotting, so changes in mental status could also signal a stroke.

Poor appetite. Like other body systems, the digestive system receives less blood when heart failure is present, which in turn causes problems with digestion. Lower cardiac output and fluid retention can lead to a tender or swollen abdomen. Heart failure patients often complain that they feel full or bloated or experience nausea or indigestion.

Irregular heartbeat. *Arrhythmia,* as this is called, describes a heart that beats too slowly, rapidly, early, or irregularly. It occurs as the heart attempts to compensate for its reduced pumping capacity. Sometimes the heartbeat speeds up to help the heart get enough blood to organs and muscles.

Several problems may cause an irregular heartbeat: a patient may have an enlarged heart, a deficiency of oxygenated blood in the heart muscle, too much pressure on the heart, or changes to the organ's electrical conduction system. Sometimes a change in the blood chemistry or *electrolytes,* such as potassium, can cause an irregular heartbeat, and your doctor will routinely check these as part of your blood tests. Be sure to tell your physician if you notice an irregular heartbeat.

Increased nighttime urination. It's common for people living with heart failure to urinate more frequently during the night. While they're lying down, blood flow to the kidneys may increase, which in turn causes the bean-shaped organs to produce more urine. Patients with severe heart failure, however, may urinate less often since their kidneys don't receive enough blood to produce urine.

Additional common symptoms. Several other symptoms are associated with heart failure, including engorged neck veins, unusual weight gain, and cool feet and hands due to poor circulation.

Are there different levels of heart failure?

Because heart failure is typically progressive, the condition is divided into stages. You may hear your doctor talk about two different methods for classifying heart failure. The first is the New York Heart Association's (NYHA) clinical classifications, which rank patients based on their degree of functionality, or how their heart failure symptoms affect day-to-day life. The second, developed by the American Heart Association (AHA) and the American College of Cardiology (ACC) in 2001, is designed to evaluate the development and progression of heart failure.

NYHA clinical classifications. Doctors still rely on this functional classification system, updated most recently in 1994, to determine the most appropriate course of therapy. The system ties symptoms to the patient's quality of life. Determining a patient's stage is a subjective assessment made by his or her doctor, and it may change frequently as symptoms improve or worsen.

> **Class 1.** People have no limitations in their physical activity. Ordinary activities don't cause undue tiredness, heart palpitations, or shortness of breath.

> **Class 2.** Patients experience mild symptoms that only slightly limit their physical activity. They're comfortable while resting, but ordinary physical activity causes fatigue, heart palpitations, or shortness of breath.

> **Class 3.** At this point, people notice a marked limitation in physical activity. While they remain comfortable at rest,

they become fatigued and short of breath and have heart palpitations even during less-than-ordinary activities.

Class 4. Patients are severely limited because they're unable to carry out any physical activity without discomfort. They have symptoms even while resting.

AHA and ACC stages of heart failure. The AHA and ACC expanded the range of classifications to include not only those with symptomatic heart failure but also those at risk of developing the condition. They did so because it is now widely known that therapeutic interventions, performed before the onset of symptoms, improve the survival rate for those afflicted with heart failure. This classification system isn't meant to replace the NYHA's but rather complement it.

The following stages may help patients understand where they fall in the progression of the condition and why they've been given a new medication, advised to undergo a surgical procedure, or encouraged to make lifestyle changes. Once a patient moves to the next stage, there's no going back, even if symptoms subside.

Stage A. During this stage, as well as stage B, the patient exhibits no symptoms. However, during stage A, the risk for developing heart failure is high for someone with one of the following predisposing factors: existing hypertension, diabetes, coronary artery disease, or metabolic syndrome; a history of rheumatic fever, alcohol abuse, or *cardiotoxic* drug therapy; or a family history of cardiomyopathy. See chapter 3 to learn about these risk factors.

Patients with stage A heart failure are strongly encouraged to exercise regularly and to stop smoking, drinking alcohol, and taking illegal drugs. Physicians treat their hypertension and lipid disorders. They also may prescribe a type of drug known as an ACE inhibitor to those who have suffered previous heart attacks or who have conditions such as high blood pressure or diabetes, and they may prescribe appropriate medications as well to people with hypertension.

Stage B. This second stage encompasses people diagnosed with heart failure, usually during an echocardiogram, but still exhibiting no symptoms. Typically, patients continue all the therapies from stage A, and they may receive a surgical consultation for a coronary artery bypass graft or valve replacement or repair. At this stage, almost all patients should receive an ACE inhibitor and a beta-blocker. Your doctor will determine what is best for your condition.

Stage C. During the third stage, heart failure has been diagnosed, and the patient is either currently experiencing symptoms or has experienced them in the past. Those symptoms include shortness of breath, fatigue, and a reduced tolerance to exercise. All the therapies from stages A and B apply. In addition, doctors may prescribe a diuretic (water pills) and digoxin. Patients in stage C should restrict salt and fluid intake and watch their weight. Also, a pacemaker or implantable cardiac defibrillator may be recommended.

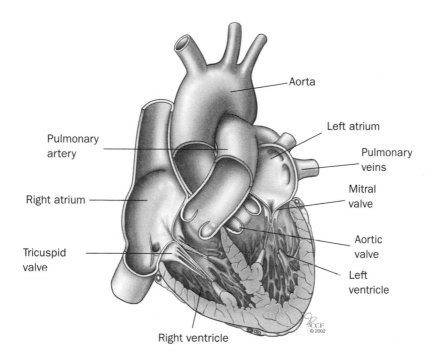

Figure 1 *Heart cross section*

Stage D. Patients experience advanced symptoms of heart failure even after receiving optimal medical care. All the therapies for stages A, B, and C apply. People with stage D heart failure need to be evaluated for the following treatments: heart transplant, ventricular assist devices, other surgery options, continuous IV infusion of inotropic drugs (which affect the force of the heart's contractions), research therapies, and even the possibility of end-of-life care. Stage D is the most severe form of heart failure and may require immediate consultation at a specialized heart failure center to determine which treatment is most appropriate.

Chapter 2

Testing for Heart Failure

If your primary care physician refers you to a *cardiologist* because he or she suspects that you have heart failure, one of the first steps is to run diagnostic tests. Such tests are critical because they help cardiologists not only make the initial diagnosis but also identify the type of heart failure you may have and select a treatment plan. Even after the diagnosis has been rendered, you'll probably continue to undergo additional tests to determine whether your condition is stable, improving, or progressing.

Prior to testing, the cardiologist will schedule an office visit where he or she performs good old-fashioned "doctoring." This first step in your heart health assessment may include the following:

- Documenting your medical history thoroughly
- Listing all your symptoms
- Recording your vital signs, such as blood pressure, temperature, and pulse
- Examining your chest by hand to estimate the size of your heart
- Ordering standard blood and urine tests to check your kidney and thyroid function, cholesterol levels, the possibility of anemia, and other things
- Listening carefully to your heart and lungs with a *stethoscope*

While primary care physicians routinely perform this latter exam, the cardiologist's trained ear hones in on a few things in particular. The doctor hears your heart filling and emptying and the valves opening and closing. He or she also listens for *rales*: crackling or gurgling sounds that indicate fluid in the lungs. In addition, the physician checks for a rapid or irregular heart rate.

MaryBeth

When MaryBeth was admitted to Cleveland Clinic late one night in January 1999, she felt as if her whole world had been turned upside down. Just the day before, she was going about her everyday tasks in one of the city's eastern suburbs: she dropped off her daughter at kindergarten and went to the grocery store. But when MaryBeth returned home and unloaded her car, she passed out.

A friend drove MaryBeth to an urgent medical care center, where the doctor performed an electrocardiogram to test her heart's electrical activity. "It was very rapid," recalls MaryBeth. "They saw something very wrong there." She was sent to a local hospital, and the next morning an echocardiogram revealed that she had an ejection fraction of only 35 percent. Late that evening, she was transferred to Cleveland Clinic.

Over the next 24 hours, MaryBeth underwent a battery of tests. When a follow-up echocardiogram showed that her ejection fraction had slipped to 20 percent, MaryBeth was sent for a cardiac catheterization. "I was extremely nervous," she says. "They had to give me a lot of Ativan because I was so antsy." The sedative helped keep her growing anxiety in check.

As the medical team inserted a catheter into a blood vessel near MaryBeth's groin and guided it to her heart, the apprehensive patient continually asked questions about the procedure and glanced at the video monitor displaying the chambers of her heart as well as her arteries. "The doctor and nurses were good at telling me what to expect," she recalls. "They told me to expect a warm sensation all the way down my leg after they injected the dye. Sure enough, a few minutes later, my leg had a warm feeling."

The echocardiogram, cardiac catheterization, and an electrophysiology study performed the next day confirmed that MaryBeth had cardiomyopathy and heart failure. Although most patients are nervous about undergoing such tests, they are invaluable for diagnosis and treatment. One week later, doctors implanted a defibrillator in MaryBeth's chest and prescribed two types of drugs: a beta-blocker *and an* ACE inhibitor. *She continues to take the medication today and leads a fulfilling life.*

How do doctors diagnose heart failure?

Thanks to advances in medical technology, cardiologists have numerous tools to help them determine not only whether patients have heart failure but also pinpoint the cause and severity of the condition. As a patient, you're likely to undergo one or more of the tests described here.

BNP blood test

The procedure: *BNP,* or *B-type natriurectic peptide,* is a substance that's secreted from the lower chambers (ventricles) of the heart in response to heart failure. The level of BNP in the circulation increases when your heart can't pump enough blood to feed your body and lowers when the condition stabilizes. Doctors use the results to diagnose heart failure, grade its severity, and monitor the effects of any treatments you're receiving.

How it's done: Your physician draws blood from a vein in your arm during an office visit, and you will probably get the results while there or within 24 hours. The test may also be conducted in the emergency room if you're in distress and doctors are trying to decide whether you have heart failure or another medical problem.

Cardiac catheterization

The procedure: During this invasive test, X-ray movies of your valves, coronary arteries, and heart chambers are taken. Diagnostic catheterization measures blood pressure inside the heart and pulmonary arteries, the level of oxygen in the blood, and the amount of *plaque* that may be built up in the arterial walls, impeding circulation. The results help cardiologists determine the best treatment options and adjust medication. You may also hear your doctor call this procedure *coronary angiography*, which refers to taking pictures of the blood vessels or coronary arteries.

How it's done: The test is typically performed in a cardiac catheterization lab. You may be sedated prior to receiving a local anesthetic, which numbs the area where a *sheath* will be placed in your artery or vein. The sheath is a small tube with a valve at the end. Next a slender, flexible tube called a *catheter* is inserted into a blood vessel in the arm or leg, then guided gently to your heart with the help of a special X-ray machine. *Contrast dye* may be injected through the catheter to help improve the definition of the X-ray images.

In addition, your doctor may conduct a heart *biopsy* during catheterization. A special catheter with snippers on the end is eased into the heart through the same sheath. The doctor is then able to obtain a small piece of tissue from your right ventricle, which is later studied under a microscope. The biopsy can help clarify several things, such as whether heart failure has been triggered by inflammation from a virus or bacteria or, in patients who have undergone a heart transplant, whether the body is rejecting the donor organ.

A basic cardiac catheterization lasts approximately a half hour, but the entire process, from preparation to recovery, may take two to four hours.

Most patients find the procedure a little uncomfortable rather than painful. The doctors use sufficient local anesthetic around the sheath entry site to numb any pain. Since you are awake throughout the procedure, if at any point you do feel pain, you can ask for more anesthetic.

Chest radiography

The procedure: A *chest X-ray* uses small amounts of radiation to make images of the structures within the chest, including the heart, blood vessels, and lungs. It shows the size of your heart and whether there is congestion in your lungs and around your heart.

How it's done: During this painless procedure, you stand or lie down on a table with your chest pressed against a boxlike piece of equipment containing X-ray film or a plate that records digital images. An X-ray tube, about six feet away, takes a picture from the back. Your doctor will probably also order a side view. During the procedure, which lasts only 15 minutes or so, the machine produces a small burst of invisible X-ray light that passes through your body onto the film, recording an image of your chest.

Echocardiogram

The procedure: Commonly called an "echo," this test uses sound waves to produce moving images of the beating heart. This is usually conducted as a painless outpatient procedure, although at times there can be some mild discomfort as the echo probe is pushed against your skin. The echo shows the size, shape, and position of your heart's structures. It also detects and measures blood flow across the heart's valves and pressure within its chambers. An echocardiogram provides much important information to your cardiologist and can be repeated over time to make comparisons.

How it's done: An echo can be performed at your doctor's office or the hospital. After you lie down on an exam table, a technician or physician will apply several small, flat, sticky patches called *electrodes* to your chest, then place a probe on your chest. You will then be asked to lie to one side, placing your body in the right position for the best images to be recorded. Before the echo probe is placed on the outside of your chest, its tip is smothered with gel that helps improve the quality of the imaging. The probe sends and receives high-frequency *ultrasound waves* that are bounced off your heart. The echocardiogram equipment translates the sound waves into pictures, which reveal abnormalities.

The technician or physician will pause the video periodically to measure the heart and all of its structures, which enables the calculation of *ejection fraction, stroke volume,* and *cardiac output.* Doctors rely on these important measurements to decide whether your heart failure is stable, improving, or progressing. During the procedure you will, at times, hear the amplified sound of your heart beating. At the end, you will be given a towel to wipe the gel off your skin.

Your physician may order a variety of echocardiograms, including one or more of the following:

Doppler echocardiography employs uses the same techniques as a regular echo but also assesses the speed and direction of blood flow. It is useful for measuring the function of the heart's valves during pumping and resting. Doppler and basic echo provide the information to determine whether a diseased heart valve should be repaired or replaced.

Transesophageal echocardiography (TEE) produes a more detailed look at the heart and often the valves by having the patient swallow a small ultrasound probe. The device's position is adjusted within the esophagus so that it sits right next to the heart. Prior to insertion, the patient's throat is sprayed with a topical anesthetic to prevent gagging. After the exam, the probe is removed.

Contrast echocardiography relies on a contrast agent injected into a vein in your arm. The agent is more efficient at bouncing sound waves back to the probe than the blood itself. Contrast echo is particularly helpful for imaging overweight patients or those with lung diseases.

Stress echocardiography helps ascertain the fitness level of your heart and lungs. It also helps diagnose coronary artery disease. First you exercise on a treadmill or stationary bike. When you can no longer continue, the echo is performed and compared with echo images taken at rest before the stress test. For those unable to exercise at all, one of several drugs can be administered intravenously to make the heart respond as though it were exercising. A healthy heart contracts more vigorously with exercise, but a region of the heart wall that doesn't contract briskly with physical activity may signal a blockage in a coronary artery.

Electrocardiogram (ECG)

The procedure: Commonly referred to as an ECG, this test records the heart's electrical activity. It gives your doctor information about your heart rate, regularity of heartbeats, and the size and position of the heart's chambers. It also shows heart damage and can help doctors decide whether drugs or devices used to regulate the heart are working.

How it's done: During the painless test, technicians will place approximately ten electrodes on your chest and extremities. These are attached to a monitor that charts electrical impulses on graph paper.

Electrophysiology (EP) study

The procedure: Similar to an ECG, this test records the electrical activity of your heart. But the EP study focuses primarily on rhythm disturbances, one of the causes of heart failure. During the test, doctors may safely reproduce your arrhythmia (such as slow or fast heartbeats) to determine the cause of the abnormal heart rhythm, its site of origin, and optimal treatment.

How it's done: While you lie on a bed, nurses will insert an intravenous line in your arm or hand to provide medications or fluids during the procedure. In addition, you'll receive medication to help you relax, although you won't be asleep. The doctor will numb your groin and insert into a nearby vein several catheters, which are then guided to your heart. These catheters sense the electrical activity in your heart and appraise your heart's conduction system.

The doctor will use a pacemaker to increase your heart rate and see your arrhythmia in action. You'll likely feel your heart beating more quickly or more slowly, and it's important to tell the physician whether you feel better or worse. If your arrhythmia occurs, the doctor may administer medications to see how you react. The EP study generally takes between two and four hours.

Magnetic resonance imaging (MRI)

The procedure: MRIs are being used more frequently in heart imaging because they offer valuable, high-resolution pictures of the heart, its vessels, and all its structures without the use of X-rays or invasive procedures. An MRI helps doctors study the size and thickness of the heart's chambers and the extent of damage caused by heart failure. MRI relies on radiofrequency waves and a very powerful magnet to create images. The use of the magnetic field means that patients with metallic implants, such as pacemakers or implantable cardiac defibrillators, can't undergo the procedure.

How it's done: MRI examinations are performed by cardiologists or radiologists who analyze and interpret the images. The noninvasive scan is performed while the patient lies on a table that's slowly moved into a long, tube-shaped device. You must lie totally still within the closed cylindrical magnet for 15 to 45 minutes while a scanner produces images of the heart from many angles.

Physicians may prescribe mild, short-acting sedatives for claustrophobic patients. In addition, newer open MRI systems have more space around the imaging table so the magnet does not completely surround the patient. Occasionally, contrast materials are given intravenously to enhance visibility of the heart's chambers and major vessels.

Multigated acquisition (MUGA) scan

The procedure: Also known as a *MUGA scan* or a *cardiac blood pool study,* this nuclear scan evaluates the pumping function of the heart's ventricles. A MUGA scan also can be used to calculate your ejection fraction. It can be performed while patients are resting or exercising during a stress test.

How it's done: Electrodes are placed on the patient's chest to record the heart's electrical activity. A small amount of a mildly radioactive isotope is injected into a vein, usually in your hand or arm, and absorbed by healthy tissue. A second injection contains a tracer that's tracked using a special camera, or *scanner,* held over your chest. (Some medical facilities may combine the two substances in one injection.) The scanner follows the isotope as it circulates through the bloodstream and into the heart and displays images of the heart in motion for analysis.

Don't let the word *radioactive* scare you: the MUGA scan is not dangerous. The isotopes are totally gone from the body within a few days.

Positron emission tomography (PET)

The procedure: Typically called a *PET scan,* this highly specialized technique uses radioactive substances to produce images as those substances function in the body. The images measure metabolic activity of the tissues, most often in the brain and heart. A cardiac PET scan provides very clear images of blood flow and how it's affected by narrow arteries and heart attack. It can help identify weakened heart muscle that may have normal function after circulation is restored.

How it's done: Just as in a MUGA scan, patients receive a short-lived radiopharmaceutical injected into a vein. They rest while the radioactive substance moves into the heart tissue, which takes approximately 30 to 90 minutes. Then patients lie on a mechanical table that eases into a doughnut-shaped scanner.

The scanner records *gamma rays* and maps the area containing the radioactive substances, enabling doctors to evaluate the heart's ongoing metabolism. This may take between 30 and 45 minutes. Your physician may request two PET scans: one performed at rest and another after administration of a pharmaceutical that alters blood flow to the heart. A radiologist performs the tests and sends the results to your physician.

What does my ejection fraction number really mean?

If you're sitting in the waiting room before your diagnostic tests, you may hear other patients throw around numbers:

"My ejection fraction is thirty-five."

"The treatment is working: my EF rose to fifty!"

In a numbers-obsessed world, where people put stock in everything from college entrance exam scores to point spreads on sporting events, it's no surprise that heart failure patients want to know their ejection fraction (EF). But what is it exactly?

Simply put, the ejection fraction is a measurement of the amount of blood pumped out of your heart during each beat. In a healthy heart, between 50 percent and 70 percent of the blood is ejected during each beat. But people with damaged hearts typically have an EF of 40 percent or less, indicating their hearts are no longer pumping efficiently. Doctors usually perform an echocardiogram to find out your EF.

Be cautioned, though, that your ejection fraction number is not precise; in fact, it may vary by 5 percent to 10 percent—even on the same day. So rather than using your EF as the only indicator of your condition, be sure to ask your doctor for his or her opinion on your overall progress. Your physician will look at many variables, including the EF, to assess your condition. It's important to remember that many patients experience no increase in their EF from their treatment. Nonetheless they feel much better, deriving great benefit from their prescribed medications together with the dietary, exercise, and lifestyle programs they embark upon.

There are, as you can see, many diagnostic tests and procedures available to help doctors accurately diagnose heart failure. Each provides a unique set of helpful information. As a result, it is quite common for cardiologists to use more than one so that they are able to build up a detailed picture of how the patient's heart is functioning.

Chapter 3

Causes of Heart Failure

Joe

In 1994 Joe was a supervisor at an aluminum plant in southern Ohio. On a warm summer evening, while attending a friend's retirement party at a VFW hall, he started feeling sick. On the way home, Joe realized that his nausea and sweating weren't just caused by a few too many celebratory beers.

"As I was driving," he recalls, "my arm hurt more. Then the pain started spreading across my chest. I knew I was

having a heart attack. I knew it. I thought I was dying at age fifty-two."

Somehow Joe made it home, nearly 90 miles away. Later that evening at the local hospital's emergency room, doctors confirmed Joe's suspicions. He'd suffered a heart attack.

Over the next three years, Joe was in and out of the hospital with chest pains and arrhythmia. "After my heart attack, the left side of my heart just stopped functioning," he says. "My heart was enlarged, and I was having trouble breathing. My family doctor just didn't know what to do anymore."

Joe came to Cleveland Clinic in September 1997 to begin aggressive treatment for heart failure. (The rest of Joe's story appears in chapter 8.) His story is not unique: coronary artery disease and heart attack are the primary causes of heart failure. But they aren't the only ones.

As we age, our eyesight and hearing often worsen, joints become inflamed, skin loses elasticity, and bones turn more brittle. No part of the human body is impervious to aging, including the heart, which loses some of its blood-pumping capability.

In addition, the chances for developing heart failure are compounded by other health issues that damage or overwork the organ. These range from persistently high blood pressure, diabetes, viruses, and hereditary conditions to unhealthy behaviors. As I've mentioned before, it's important that your doctor understand the root cause of your heart failure in order to treat it properly. This chapter reviews some of the major causes of heart failure.

Coronary Artery Disease (CAD)

When the arteries that supply blood and oxygen to the heart muscle become diseased, heart failure can ensue. Nutrients are delivered to the heart muscle by its own set of arteries attached to the outside of the heart muscle. *Coronary artery disease* develops when the arteries' inner lining breaks down and the walls thicken. Whereas a child's arterial walls are smooth and elastic, aging tubular vessels become streaked with fat. In turn, the damaged arteries release chemicals that make their walls tacky. Plaque, a material made up of cholesterol, fatty deposits, and other substances, builds up in the walls, eventually narrowing the opening and restricting the flow of blood. We call this *atherosclerosis,* but it's commonly referred to as *hardening of the arteries.*

A plaque can rupture, and a blot clot forms suddenly, leading to total occlusion of an artery. This generally results in chest pain and requires emergency treatment. A 50 percent blockage due to the buildup of plaque, but causing no symptoms, can suddenly become a 100 percent blockage due to the blood clot and lead to a full-blown heart attack.

A heart starved of oxygen and nutrients due to reduced circulation can't function properly. The organ has difficulty responding to increased activity, which may produce chest pain (*angina*) and other symptoms of heart disease.

How common is coronary artery disease?

According to the National Heart, Lung, and Blood Institute, approximately 13 million people in the United States have coronary artery disease. It's also the leading cause of death in both men and women, with more than 500,000 Americans dying annually from CAD. Unfortunately, some degree of arterial narrowing is normal as we age. And almost half of all patients don't know they have coronary artery disease until a fatal event strikes. For this reason, doctors assess each patient for associated risk factors and encourage patients to adopt a healthy lifestyle.

What are the symptoms of coronary artery disease?

Angina is the most prevalent indication of CAD. People complain of heaviness, pressure, burning, or numbness in their chests. Sometimes they dismiss it as indigestion or heartburn. Other signs may include shortness of breath, weakness, palpitations, nausea, or sweating. Symptoms typically occur with exertion but can happen with minimal activity, mental or emotional stress, and even at rest.

Heart Attack

Each year, more than 1 million Americans suffer heart attacks, also called *myocardial infarctions*. They happen when a coronary artery becomes completely blocked, halting the flow of blood to the heart.

Arteries become obstructed when plaque builds up. The hard shell of plaque may crack, and the body's responds by sending *blood platelet cells* to the area to assist in clotting. Blood clots then form around the plaque. If a blood clot totally blocks the artery, the much-needed oxygen supply is cut off from the region of the heart nearest the blockage. This lack of oxygen and nutrients leads to a death of heart muscle cells. The term *myocardial infarction* translates as "death of the tissue [infarction] in the heart muscle [myocardial]."

Can the heart heal after a heart attack?

Just as the body heals other wounds, it takes approximately eight weeks following a myocardial infarction for the heart muscle to heal and form scar tissue. But scarred tissue isn't as pliant as healthy heart muscle, and it can diminish the heart's efficiency. To what degree the pumping capacity is impaired depends on the size and location of the scar tissue.

Because of the lingering damage to the heart, a heart attack significantly increases a person's chances of developing heart failure. According to a 2006 report by the American Heart Association, approximately 22 percent of men and 46 percent of women who have suffered heart attacks will develop heart failure within six years.

Is cardiac arrest the same as a heart attack?

Cardiac arrest is often mistakenly referred to as a heart attack. Cardiac arrest happens when the electrical system of the heart unexpectedly malfunctions. As a result, the heart can

Sudden Cardiac Death: The Silent Killer

Sudden cardiac death (SCD) occurs when the heart beats so abnormally that it stops pumping blood. Some patients experience a racing heartbeat or dizziness, alerting the sufferer to a problem. Typically, SCD strikes without warning symptoms and can lead to death within minutes unless it's treated immediately.

SCD is the leading cause of natural death in the United States, killing about 325,000 adults annually, according to the Cleveland Clinic Heart and Vascular Institute. Although it often occurs without warning, it can be treated and reversed if the following emergency actions are taken within minutes:

1. Call 911.

2. Perform *CPR (cardiopulmonary resuscitation)* on the victim to keep blood and oxygen circulating until medical help arrives.

3. Defibrillate the person if you have access to an ambulatory external defibrillator. This quick delivery of an electric shock returns an abnormal heart rhythm to normal.

4. Get the person advanced care at a hospital to treat and prevent future cardiac problems.

stop entirely, slow down, or beat so irregularly and quickly that it becomes an ineffective pump, unable to deliver blood throughout the body. By contrast, a heart attack occurs when one or more coronary arteries are blocked, preventing the heart from getting enough oxygen-rich blood. There-fore, the heart is damaged.

Cardiomyopathy

If the heart muscle has been damaged and the possibil-ity of arterial blockage or restricted blood flow has been eliminated, then the likely cause is *cardiomyopathy*. Simply put, cardiomyopathy refers to a host of diseases or prob-lems intrinsic to the heart muscle. Sometimes it occurs without any known reason, when it is known as *idiopathic cardiomyopathy*.

Often the heart muscle becomes damaged through the action of a virus, alcohol or drug abuse, or metabolic disease. In addition, cardiomyopathy can be associated with genetic disorders, obesity, pregnancy, radiation, chemotherapy, and others. Whatever the cause, the disease accounts for up to half of all heart failure cases.

With so many causes, how can cardiomyopathy be classified?

There are three primary types of cardiomyopathy: *dilated, hypertrophic,* and *restrictive*. A fourth type, *arrhythmogenic right ventricular cardiomyopathy,* is less common. Most forms of cardiomyopathy can be inherited; however, our ability to perform and interpret genetic testing remains quite limited.

Dilated cardiomyopathy (DCM). In DCM, the most frequent form of cardiomyopathy, one or both of the heart's chambers enlarge (dilate). You may also hear doctors call the condition *cardiac dilatation*. As the heart becomes enlarged, it pumps out less blood; consequently, more blood remains in the distended ventricle after each heartbeat. In many cases, DCM is discovered by an abnormal ECG or echo or a sudden loss of consciousness.

In most cases, the cause of dilated cardiomyopathy remains unknown. However, some factors can contribute to the condition. These include genetics, viral infections, autoimmune diseases, and alcohol abuse. Very rarely, women in the middle to late stages of pregnancy or who are postpartum can develop cardiomyopathy.

Hypertrophic cardiomyopathy (HCM). Hypertrophic cardiomyopathy affects 1 in 500 people, causing the heart muscle to thicken, or hypertrophy. Associated findings also include left ventricular stiffness, changes in the mitral valve, and cellular changes.

HCM has two types: obstructive and nonobstructive. It is considered obstructive if the wall between the two ventricles (the septum) becomes enlarged and impedes the blood flow out of the left ventricle to the aorta. In response, the ventricles pump more aggressively to overcome the blockage.

In patients with nonobstructive HCM, the thickened heart muscle doesn't interfere with circulation. The heart may contract normally, but it fills improperly between heartbeats so that blood backs up in the veins leading to the heart. This in turn causes high blood pressure in the lungs, or *secondary pulmonary hypertension.*

Hypertrophic cardiomyopathy can be inherited or acquired. Those who inherit HCM have an abnormality in the gene that codes characteristics of the heart muscle. Although hypertrophy may be present at birth, it usually shows up during adolescence or early adulthood. It is important to note, however, that some people with the gene defect never develop HCM. In addition, hypertrophic cardiomyopathy often results from aging and high blood pressure.

Initial symptoms may be very nonspecific and include shortness of breath, dizziness, or lightheadedness with exertion and heart fluttering or palpitations. Teenagers and young adults who experience any of these symptoms during athletic events or with exertion should see their physicians for testing. If there is a family history of hypertrophic cardiomyopathy, please discuss this with your doctor, who may advise evaluation by a cardiologist.

Restrictive cardiomyopathy. Restrictive cardiomyopathy occurs when the heart resists filling properly because the ventricles are stiff. The heart's pumping strength usually remains normal. This is a very rare and uncommon form of cardiomyopathy. It is sometimes confused with other medical conditions because it is difficult to diagnose and requires a comprehensive evaluation.

This uncommon form of the disease may be caused by abnormal scarring of the heart tissue (*fibrosis*) or an unexplained phenomenon in which the heart relaxes between beats. It also may occur when certain substances, including iron or proteins, enter the heart muscle or because of rare metabolic disorders.

Arrhythmogenic right ventricular cardiomyopathy (ARVC). In ARVC, heart muscle gets replaced by scar tissue and fat, with the right ventricle being most affected. ARVC often appears in patches, so diseased areas may be bordered by healthy muscle. As the condition progresses, the right side of the heart dilates, the muscle deteriorates, and thin layers of fat and fibrous tissue form.

ARVC is usually associated with an irregular heartbeat (arrhythmia), which can cause lightheadedness or even passing out (spells that doctors refer to as *syncope*). The exact cause of ARVC remains unknown, but evidence shows that it may be hereditary.

High Blood Pressure (Hypertension)

About 50 million American adults—or 1 in 3—have chronically elevated blood pressure (*hypertension*), according to the Heart and Vascular Institute at Cleveland Clinic. Why is that so disturbing? Because it puts those people at risk for heart disease, stroke, and heart failure.

The risks are quite real: a 2006 report by the American Heart Association states that 75 percent of heart failure cases are preceded by high blood pressure. And people with high blood pressure are two to three times more likely to develop heart failure.

Blood pressure measures the force of blood pushing against the blood vessel walls with each heartbeat. When a doctor or nurse places a blood pressure cuff on your arm and listens with a stethoscope, a special meter records two numbers: your systolic and diastolic blood pressure. Systolic measures the amount of pressure each time the heart contracts, while diastolic measures the pressure when the heart is at rest. A normal reading should be less than 120/80 (systolic/diastolic) mm Hg (millimeters of mercury).

When your blood pressure is higher than 120/80, your heart has to pump more vigorously to keep your blood circulating. If the heart works too hard, then heart failure ensues.

Arrhythmia

Put simply, an arrhythmia is an abnormal heart rhythm. The heart beats too rapidly, too slowly, or irregularly and may not be able to pump enough blood to sustain the body.

The heart is an amazing machine, synchronizing its rhythm with a built-in electrical system. An electrical impulse triggered at the *sinus node* (also called the *sinoatrial node*) indicates the start of each heartbeat. This small mass of tissue, located in the right atrium, generates the electrical signals that dictate the rate and rhythm of your heartbeat. Accordingly, it is often referred to as the heart's natural pacemaker.

The impulse extends through the walls of the right and left atriums, causing the chambers to contract and force blood into the ventricles. Next the impulse travels to the *atrioventricular (AV) node.* Think of the AV node as a link set up so that electrical impulses can pass from the atriums to the ventricles. From there, the signal moves through a trail of fibers that sends it into the ventricles, making them contract and pump blood out to the lungs and body.

When doctors take your pulse, they're measuring your heart rate, or the number of times it beats in one minute. A normal resting heart rate is between 50 and 100 beats per minute. If you have arrhythmia, your heart may beat more slowly than 60 beats or more quickly than 100 beats per minute.

What causes arrhythmia?

There are many causes of abnormal heartbeats. Some are due to problems with the heart, such as coronary artery disease, high blood pressure, heart attack, or valve disorders. Others are caused by outside forces, such as caffeine, nicotine, alcohol, diet pills, or cold medicines. Shock and stress may also trigger arrhythmias.

Can arrhythmia cause sudden cardiac arrest?

Many arrhythmias go unnoticed by those who have them. Others cause shortness of breath, heart palpitations, a pounding in the chest, or dizziness. Abnormal heartbeats can often be treated with medication or lifestyle changes. But sometimes they are severe enough to cause heart failure. An abnormal heart rhythm is the most common cause of the abrupt loss of heart function known as *sudden cardiac arrest.* Your chances of experiencing SCA, also called *sudden cardiac death,* increase if you've previously suffered a heart attack or have coronary artery disease or heart failure. In fact, people with heart failure are six to nine times more likely to experience arrhythmias that may lead to sudden cardiac arrest, according to the Cleveland Clinic Heart and Vascular Institute.

Valve Disease and Infection

Your heart has four sets of flaplike valves (the mitral, tricuspid, aortic, and pulmonic), which are responsible for ensuring blood flows in only one direction through your heart. Valve disease is present when one or more of the pairs don't function correctly because of either *valvular stenosis* (obstruction) or *valvular insufficiency* (leakage).

Valvular stenosis is a narrowing of the valves. The tissue that make up the flaps becomes stiff, thereby narrowing the valve opening and reducing the amount of blood that can flow through it. If the *stenotic* valve is only mildly affected, the heart can usually function adequately. But the valve can taper to such a degree that the body doesn't receive an adequate blood supply, and heart failure ensues.

Valvular insufficiency occurs when the flaps don't close completely, allowing blood to leak backward. The reverse flow is called *regurgitant flow.* You may also hear people refer to valvular insufficiency as having a "leaky valve."

How does someone develop valve disease?

People can be born with valve disease or acquire it later in life. Sometimes the cause remains unknown; other times it's caused by coronary artery disease, heart attack, cardiomyopathy, hypertension, or other conditions. In addition, infection is often to blame. Endocarditis and rheumatic fever are two common infections that can cause valve disease.

Endocarditis is a serious, sometimes life-threatening infection that occurs when bacteria enters your bloodstream and stick to the surface of your heart valves, causing growths, holes, or scarring of the valve tissue. *Rheumatic fever* is an inflammatory disease that can develop after an infection with streptococcus bacteria, such as strep throat and scarlet fever. It can lead to rheumatic heart disease, which causes the heart valves to inflame, narrow, or leak or the flaps to stick together or scar.

Congenital Heart Defects

Congenital heart defects, which develop while the fetus is growing in the uterus, affect one or more structures of the heart or blood vessels and are present in approximately 8 to 10 births out of 1,000, according to the Cleveland Clinic Heart and Vascular Institute. Sometimes symptoms arise at birth or in childhood, other times not until the afflicted person reaches adulthood.

Essentially, the heart's structures don't form correctly: parts may be missing altogether or misplaced, or they may be too narrow or big. The Adult Congenital Heart Disease Association says that there are more than 30 different kinds of congenital heart defects. The most common ones affecting adults are valve defects (discussed earlier in this chapter), atrial and ventricular septal defects, and patent foramen ovale.

An *atrial septal defect* is a hole in the muscular wall between the left and right atriums, the heart's upper chambers. If the hole is large, then blood from the left atrium travels back to the right atrium and is then pumped back into the lungs. This forces the heart to work harder.

A *ventricular septal defect* is a hole in the septum separating the heart's two lower chambers. In a healthy heart, the pressure in the right ventricle is lower than in the left one. If the hole is large, blood can travel between the two ventricles, which alters the pressure in each and makes the heart function less efficiently.

Patent foramen ovale refers to a small hole in the atrial septum that's critical for fetal circulation. A baby in the womb receives blood from its mother's placenta. The blood flows through the umbilical cord to the fetus. The blood then moves directly from the right to the left side of the baby's heart through the foramen ovale, bypassing the lungs.

Typically, the foramen ovale closes when a baby is born. If it doesn't, the defect is called a patent foramen ovale. The hole often acts like a flap, opening when there's pressure in the heart. If the pressure is strong enough, blood can move directly between the right and left atria.

According to the Cleveland Clinic Heart and Vascular Institute, approximately 500,000 people in the United States grow into adulthood with congenital heart disease, and that number increases by about 20,000 annually. As those adults' hearts work harder to compensate for the defects, they are at risk for heart failure.

Other Causes

Many other conditions can contribute to heart failure by placing excessive strain on the heart. These include severe anemia, an overactive thyroid, chronic kidney disease, diabetes, severe lung disease, and obesity. In addition, viruses can attack the heart muscle, leaving it weakened and susceptible to failure. For example, *myocarditis,* an inflammation of the heart, is a rare disorder usually caused by viral, bacterial, or parasitic infections.

Chapter 4

Treatments for Heart Failure

There are many options for treating patients with heart failure today that did not exist 60, 40, or even 20 years ago. Those range from prescribing a variety of medications that help the heart function to performing heart transplantation surgery.

According to the American Heart Association, approximately 95,000 valve replacements were performed in 2003. Some values replacements are replaced with mechanical valves made from plastic, carbon, or metal. Other are biological valves, constructed from animal tissue (called a *xenograft*) or from a donated human heart (called an *allograft* or *homograft*), as in Greg's case.

Greg

Greg was born with aortic stenosis. His aortic valve was narrow, preventing it from opening properly and hindering the flow of blood from the left ventricle to the aorta. This created extra work for the ventricle. It eventually thickened, and his heart began to fail.

Like many people with this congenital heart valve abnormality, Greg remained symptom free until adulthood. As a child, he rode bikes and skateboards and kept up with all his friends. Even at age 26, Greg remained active. He worked for a telecommunications company, climbing poles to install residential phone lines, and he played indoor soccer.

"I never noticed my bad valve until I started feeling weird and sick and ended up in the hospital with heart failure," says Greg. His decline happened gradually starting in 1998. During the spring and summer, he tired easily and sweated frequently. "I just thought I was out of shape," he says. "Then I got really sick."

In October Greg suffered from flulike symptoms: he lost his appetite, slept a lot, and had bouts of vomiting and diarrhea. Greg went to the hospital, where he was treated with antibiotics for pneumonia and sent home. But his symptoms didn't subside. Greg was then admitted to the hospital. Doctors ran several tests, including a blood workup and a transesophageal echocardiogram.

"They realized that my heart was enlarged, my aortic valve was shot, and my EF was fifteen percent," Greg recalls. "I was so sick that I didn't even know where I was at that point. I lost

about three weeks." Greg was transferred to the heart failure intensive care unit at Cleveland Clinic in November.

In early December, Greg underwent heart valve surgery, a common solution for patients with advanced valve disease. Cardiac surgeons replaced his aortic valve with a homograft and repaired his tricuspid valve, which had deteriorated due to heart failure. The repair was made with a Cosgrove-Edwards annuloplasty ring, *named after Cleveland Clinic heart surgeon Delos M. Cosgrove, who pioneered minimally invasive heart valve surgery in the mid-1990s, and Edwards Lifesciences, the company that manufactures the ring. The device supports and tightens Greg's tricuspid valve at the point where the flaps are anchored.*

Greg remained in the intensive care unit for approximately five days after surgery. He had some complications, including fluid retention and abnormal heart rhythms. But medication cleared up those problems. When Greg was released from the clinic, his ejection fraction had doubled to 30 percent.

Today Greg works 12-hour days on two jobs, remodeling homes and testing wireless connections for a telecommunications company. He also plays with his two young children and does yard work. He takes a beta-blocker and a blood pressure medication daily.

Greg is grateful for the surgical procedures and medication that allow him to live longer with his congenital valve defect. And he offers a hopeful message to others in the same situation: "It's not as big a deal as you think it is," he says. "Be concerned, but don't worry too much. It's 2007, not the 1940s. If it had been sixty years ago, I'd probably be dead. But today there are options."

Aren't all heart problems fatal?

Greg's story highlights the importance of receiving proper diagnosis and treatment. The operation to replace his aortic valve essentially reversed his heart failure and allowed him to live a normal and active life. Without surgery, Greg would not have survived. Heart failure can be stabilized or even reversed in many cases.

What kinds of treatments are there for heart failure?

This chapter presents an overview of the most common treatments available today, including medication, cardiac devices, and surgical procedures. Many patients with heart failure will receive more than one treatment at some point.

Medication

Medical therapy has advanced dramatically in the treatment of heart failure. Because the condition's cause was unknown for so many years, patients often weren't diagnosed until its later stages. At that point, their circulatory system and lungs were quite congested, so they were given diuretics to decrease excess fluid. Beyond that, there weren't many choices.

Even a decade ago, the typical treatment relied on three main classes of drugs: *diuretics* to rid the body of surplus fluids, *digoxin* to improve the heart's pumping ability, and *ACE inhibitors* to increase blood flow. But now *beta-blockers* and other medications have joined the growing list of pharmaceuticals that help heart failure patients.

It is important to work closely with your cardiologist to determine which drugs work best for you. While medication can't cure heart failure, it can help relieve your symptoms and improve your condition. Researchers at Cleveland Clinic and other medical facilities continue to investigate new *inotropic, vasodilating,* and diuretic drugs.

What kinds of medication are prescribed to treat heart failure?

A healthy person might take a daily multivitamin and perhaps the occasional aspirin to relieve a headache or muscle relaxant to soothe a sore body. But people living with heart failure often pop a half dozen pills or more as part of their daily regimen. This is a partial list of the classes of medications typically given to heart failure patients.

Angiotensin converting enzyme (ACE) inhibitors. This class of drugs dilates blood vessels to reduce blood pressure and increase the amount of blood pumped by the heart. ACE inhibitors also prevent the body from generating damaging substances (*angiotensin II*) as a consequence of heart failure. A variety of ACE inhibitors are commonly used to treat heart failure, and their use is based on extensive evidence from clinical trials. (See "Clinical Trials for Heart Failure Options" on page 62.)

Aldosterone inhibitors. *Aldosterone* is a hormone that regulates your salt and water balance. Aldosterone inhibitors, which are typically prescribed only to patients with advanced heart failure, block the hormone from causing the buildup of salt and water. Two aldosterone inhibitors that are commonly prescribed are spironolactone (brand names include Aldactone and Spironol) and eplerenone (brand names include Inspra).

Anticoagulants. Anticoagulants, which prevent the blood from clotting, are commonly used for patients with an abnormal heart rhythm (atrial fibrillation), a known blood clot in the heart, severe heart muscle weakness, or a history of stroke. They may be administered intravenously, as is the case with heparin, or orally. Warfarin (brand name: Coumadin) is a popular oral anticoagulant.

Angiotensin II receptor blockers (ARBs). This class of medication functions much as do ACE inhibitors, lowering blood pressure, improving blood flow, and preventing the actions of angiotensin II. ARBs are usually given to patients who can't tolerate ACE inhibitors.

Beta-blockers. Beta-blockers slow the heart rate, reduce blood pressure, lower the production of harmful substances produced in response to heart failure, and improve the heart's ability to relax. Commonly prescribed beta-blockers include bispropolol (brand names include Zebeta), metoprolol succinate (Toprol-XL), and carvedilol (Coreg).

Calcium channel blockers. Calcium channel blockers treat chest pain, arrhythmias, and high blood pressure. By influencing how calcium moves in the heart's cells and blood vessels, calcium channel blockers relax blood vessels, increase the supply of blood and oxygen to the heart, and reduce the cardiac workload. Two common medications used safely in patients with heart failure include amlodipine (brand name: Norvasc) and felodipine (Plendil).

Digoxin. This medication helps a damaged or weak heart pump more efficiently so that more blood travels through the body. In addition, digoxin improves blood circulation and slows the heart rate. Some brand names include Lanoxin, Lanoxicaps, and Digitek.

Diuretics. Commonly called "water pills," diuretics prevent the body from retaining too much salt by passing it in urine. That reduces swelling and makes it easier for your heart to pump. There are many diuretics on the market, including furosemide (brand name: Lasix), bumetanide (Bumex), and torsemide (Demadex). There are several types of diuretics, each with its own mechanism of action. Sometimes it may be necessary to take more than one type to ensure maximum effect.

Mineral supplements. Heart failure patients are often encouraged to take potassium and magnesium supplements to replace those minerals, which may be lost through increased urination as a result of diuretics.

Vasodilators. These help lower blood pressure by relaxing arterial blood vessels, thereby lessening the workload on the heart. Vasodilators are often used in tandem with drugs called *nitrates,* which relax the veins. The vasodilator-nitrate combination is typically given to patients who can't take an ACE inhibitor or angiotensin II receptor blocker or to those who need extra medication to control their heart failure. A clinical trial has shown that the combination of hydralazine and nitrates (brand name BiDil), when added to ACE inhibitors and beta-blockers, can provide additional benefits for African-Americans with moderate and severe heart failure.

Cardiac Devices

The development of the pacemaker and implantable defibrillator (ICD) has revolutionized the outcomes and quality of life of heart failure patients. Several implantable cardiac devices are used to help the heart function, including the following.

Cardiac resynchronization therapy (CRT)

CRT, also called *biventricular pacing,* treats the delay in ventricular contractions that occurs in some heart failure patients. The minimally invasive procedure doesn't require surgeons to open the chest; instead a small, battery-powered device is surgically implanted under the skin. Typically the procedure only requires the use of a local anesthetic. Two or three wires are threaded into the heart through veins by a catheter.

The implanted CRT sends a low current of electrical energy through the wires to the ventricles, causing them to contract simultaneously. By restoring proper timing of the heart's contractions, the heart fills with blood and works more efficiently. Some patients at risk for sudden cardiac death receive a *CRT-D* device, which includes a built-in defibrillator.

Implantable cardiac defibrillators (ICDs)

An *implantable cardiac defibrillator* is used for people with heart failure, cardiomyopathy, or irregular heartbeats. Also known simply as a defibrillator, the surgically placed electronic device continually monitors a patient's heart rhythm. If it detects an abnormality, the ICD gently shocks the heart muscle to restore a normal rhythm. The shock is generally unexpected and may be uncomfortable—even painful—but it's very brief.

An ICD consists of wires (*leads*) and a generator. The wires monitor the heart's rhythm and deliver the energy to restore the rhythm, while the generator holds the battery and a tiny computer that receives the information from the leads. There are several types of implantable defibrillators. With a *single-chamber ICD*, a lead is attached in the right ventricle. With a *dual-chamber ICD*, leads are connected to the right atrium and the right ventricle. With a *biventricular ICD*, leads are affixed in the right atrium and both ventricles.

Defibrillators are typically implanted with a minimally invasive approach. A small incision is made under the collarbone, and leads are guided to your heart through a vein.

Then the generator is slipped under the skin in your upper chest, and the leads are attached to it.

Ventricular assist devices

Ventricular assist devices mechanically help maintain the pumping ability for hearts that can no longer work effectively without assistance. Because heart failure patients typically incur greater weakness on the left side, they often receive a *left ventricular assist device,* also called an *LVAD.* But some patients instead require a *right ventricular assist device* (*RVAD*) or a combination of the two (*biventricular assist device,* or *BiVAD*).

In the United States, total artificial hearts can also be implanted as a bridge to transplant for patients with severe left and right heart failure. These devices require that the patient remains in the hospital until a suitable donor heart is found. Portable drivers are being developed that will allow patients with total artificial hearts to be discharged from hospital. This technology is currently available in Europe.

You may hear your doctor refer to ventricular assist devices as a "bridge to transplant." Patients waiting for a heart transplant often remain on the list for a while before a suitable donor heart becomes available. LVADs and RVADs can be invaluable for people whose hearts have deteriorated during the wait. They may be used for weeks or even months. For some end-stage heart failure patients who aren't transplant candidates, LVADs are permanent therapies.

Most ventricular assist devices include a pump, which is usually implanted in the abdomen. Tubes are attached to the left ventricle (to carry blood to the LVAD) and the aorta (to carry blood away from the LVAD). Internal valves assure one-way blood flow through the system. When the pump fills with blood, sensors alert the device to send blood through the tube on the aorta to the rest of the body.

Another tube is passed from the internal pump to the surface of the skin and attached to an external control system. It provides power for the device and displays messages about its status. The controller can be worn in a holster under the patient's arm or in a waist pack. Permanent LVADs are rapidly improving, and more patients with advanced heart failure are now living extended and productive lives with mechanical circulatory support devices.

Other devices. Your doctor may recommend another device, such as an *intra-aortic balloon pump (IABP)* or a *pacemaker.* The first features a pump connected to a balloon device that is inserted in the aorta to provide temporary assistance to the heart. The balloon inflates and deflates and is synchronized by the patient's own heartbeat. It reduces the work required from the weakened heart. An IABP is used to stabilize and improve the condition of critically ill hospitalized patients. If the person needs the device indefinitely, a more durable pump can be implanted.

Pacemakers monitor the heartbeat and deliver small, imperceptible electrical charges to stimulate the heartbeat if needed. Pacemakers usually treat abnormally slow heartbeats. A specialized pacemaker discussed earlier in this chapter, the biventricular pacemaker, provides cardiac resynchronization therapy (CRT).

Surgical Treatments

While surgery isn't used very often for patients with heart failure, it's a good choice for some. When medical management and lifestyle changes aren't enough to keep heart failure from progressing, physicians have four main surgical options.

Coronary artery bypass graft (CABG)

CABG surgery is an option when a coronary artery becomes blocked or there's so much plaque buildup that not enough blood flows through the coronary arteries to feed the heart. During the procedure, the surgeon makes an incision in your breastbone (sternum) to access the heart. Then the blocked arteries are bypassed using blood vessel grafts to reestablish normal cardiac blood flow. The grafts are typically taken from the patient's own arteries and veins in the chest, leg, or arm.

Bypass surgery is one of the most common open-heart operations: in 2003, approximately 467,000 of these procedures were performed in the United States, according to the National Center for Health Statistics. Surgery generally takes between three and five hours, depending on how many arteries need repair.

Valve replacement surgery

Valve replacement may be considered if heart failure is caused by a defective or diseased heart valve, as was the case with Greg, whom you met earlier in this chapter. During traditional heart valve surgery, a surgeon makes an incision in your sternum to reach the heart, then repairs or replaces the damaged valve(s). The mitral valve requires more surgeries than the other three pairs, followed by the aortic and tricuspid valves.

There are several types of valve-related procedures. During a *commissurotomy*, fused valve flaps are separated to widen the valve opening. In a *decalcification* procedure, calcium deposits are cleaned off the flaps so they become more flexible and close properly. If the valve ring, or *annulus*, is too wide, it can be reshaped or tightened by sewing a ring around it. (Greg had this type of repair performed on his tricuspid valve.) In addition, surgeons may patch holes in the flaps.

As the name suggests, valve replacement substitutes defective valves with mechanical or donor ones. Mechanical valves may be plastic or metal. Valves may be obtained from human donors or constructed from animal tissue.

Left ventricular reconstruction surgery

Left ventricular reconstruction surgery is an option for some patients with heart failure. It's also known as the *Dor procedure* after Dr. Vincent Dor, who wrote many articles on the surgery he pioneered in the 1980s. During the operation, doctors

Clinical Trials for Heart Failure Options

Much debate can occur when a medical team is considering CABG or left ventricular reconstruction surgery. A clinical trial is currently being conducted worldwide to determine the best surgical options for people with coronary artery disease and heart failure. For more information on numerous heart failure trials, visit *ClinicalTrials.gov,* an online service of the U.S. National Institutes of Health.

remove scar tissue and aneurysms that may have developed after a heart attack in the left ventricle. In addition, the chamber often loses its elliptical shape, so surgeons return it to a more normal shape. This helps improve heart function.

To begin, the surgeon opens the sternum, then makes a small incision in the left ventricle. He or she locates the dead or scarred tissue and separates it from healthy tissue with stitches. If there's a significant amount of dead tissue, it may be removed and replaced with a patch. Then the surgeon closes the outside of the ventricle and reinforces it with more stitches.

Heart transplantation

Heart transplantation, perhaps the most serious surgical procedure for correcting heart failure, is considered when other treatments have been exhausted or ruled out. Candidates are screened carefully, then are placed on a transplant waiting list. In 2004, 2,016 heart transplants were performed in the United States according to the American Heart Association. Cleveland Clinic began cardiac transplantations in 1984 and is one of only three centers to have carried out more than 1,000 of the operations. In 2007, the clinic performed 61 heart transplants.

Simply put, transplantation entails replacing the patient's damaged heart with a healthy one acquired from a donor who has been declared brain-dead. The procedure typically lasts between four and eight hours. Patients are connected to a heart-lung machine that does the work of those organs during the surgery. The heart is removed, the donor heart is put in its place, and the major blood vessels are reattached. (For more information on donor hearts, see "The Fundamentals of Organ Donation" in chapter 9.)

PART II

Patient Stories

Chapter 5

Heart Transplant: Dan's Story

"I'm alive! I feel as if I've been given a divine gift, and I feel great thanks to an organ donor, friends, family, God, and a special group of people at Cleveland Clinic."

— Dan, recipient of a heart transplant in 2005, at age 45

When I was first introduced to Dan, I thought, "This is a very sick man." I met him in early October 2004, when he came to the clinic with advanced heart failure due to familial dilated cardiomyopathy. I immediately scheduled consultations with other medical specialists, including a neurologist, lung specialist, and gastroenterologist.

It was clear that Dan needed a heart transplant, but his was a complex case—so many other factors, so many medical complications, so much more to his story. A story that started years before he walked into my office.

Dan's Story: Diagnosed with a Muscle-Wasting Disease

In 1991 Dan was an energetic outdoorsman living in the rolling hills of southwestern Pennsylvania. "I had always been a very physical person. I exercised and lifted weights," he says. "I was a tree cutter and climber by trade." But at just age 31, he noticed that he was gradually losing strength. He increased his workouts, even trying cross-training, but he continued to feel weaker.

Dan visited his family doctor, who ran urine tests and ordered an electromyogram to measure the electrical impulses of his muscles at rest and during contraction, as well as a muscle tissue biopsy. The results were sent to the Johns Hopkins Hospital in Baltimore, which diagnosed Dan with Becker's muscular dystrophy.

Becker's muscular dystrophy, an inherited disorder, causes a slow, progressive deterioration of muscles, particularly in the legs and the pelvis. The gene for Becker's muscular dystrophy is located on the X chromosome. Because women have two X chromosomes, if one carries the defective gene, the other compensates, so women sufferers typically experience much milder symptoms. Men possess both one X chromosome and one Y chromosome—the male sex chromosome. A man who inherits the mutation will develop Becker's.

Genetic testing revealed that Dan inherited the disorder from his mother, who was a carrier for the condition. Dan's symptoms appeared unusually late: according to the U.S. National Library of Medicine at the National Institutes of Health, Becker's muscular dystrophy typically announces itself around age 12, and by the age of 30, most men are no longer able to walk.

Despite the delayed onset, the debilitating disorder took its toll on Dan over the next decade. He lost strength in his legs and arms. His grip weakened, making work as a tree cutter very difficult. "The doctors told me that if I kept doing this job, the tissue teardown was going to accelerate, and the muscular dystrophy would advance a lot quicker," he recalls.

After a lot of soul searching, Dan decided there was a way he could stay in a job close to nature without the added physical strain. He earned a college degree and went to work for a state university as a researcher and part-time instructor focusing on natural resources in forests.

Muscular dystrophy attacks the heart

Dan's muscular dystrophy didn't affect only his limbs. "It went after my heart muscle the most," he says. "It slowly just killed my heart." He developed dilated cardiomyopathy and began medication through a Pittsburgh hospital. Dan received drugs to lower his blood pressure and prevent a heart attack. He also took a diuretic, digoxin, and a potassium supplement.

By the summer of 2002, Dan was referred to Johns Hopkins for a heart transplant, but he wasn't sick enough yet to land on the transplant list. "They told me I had three to five years left on my heart," remembers Dan. It was an accurate diagnosis.

Throughout 2004, Dan suffered from recurrent pneumonia. "My heart was so weak, it couldn't make my lungs work right," he says. That's when Dan came to my office for help, and I realized that it would take a team of physicians to chart his medical course. He was admitted to Cleveland Clinic several times between October 2004 and February 2005 for pneumonia and complications from heart failure. Dan also received an implanted electronic pacemaker to regulate his heartbeats.

Meanwhile, I consulted with a neurologist to decide whether the overall muscle deterioration would shorten his lifespan so significantly that a heart transplant would be moot. Because of Dan's bouts with pneumonia, I worked alongside a lung specialist. Were his chest wall muscles so compromised that he'd be likely to die from respiratory problems prior to the transplant or shortly thereafter? Ultimately the medical team decided that we could stabilize his condition and prepare him for a transplant. He very nearly didn't make it.

Hitting rock bottom

Dan remembers Presidents' Day 2005 clearly: "I was sitting at home in my easy chair watching TV, and I couldn't breathe. Everything changed right then and there—*bam!* I could tell. I told my wife to call the ambulance."

Dan was transported to a small hospital eight miles from his house. There, emergency room doctors stabilized him and called me. Dan was in severe heart failure, so I had him transferred to the clinic. It was a crash-and-burn fire drill trying to keep him alive.

Within two days, Dan received three mechanical assist devices to help his weakened heart pump more efficiently. He got an intra-aortic balloon pump and a left ventricular assist device (LVAD). While many forms of heart failure predominantly affect the left ventricle, Dan's entire heart was weakened because of his muscular dystrophy, so surgeons also implanted a right ventricular assist device (RVAD).

Without these devices, Dan would have died within 24 hours. "I was in pretty bad shape," he says stoically. He doesn't remember much after being admitted, for Dan was heavily medicated during much of the two months or so that he relied on the mechanical assist devices. But his wife, Brenda, has vivid memories.

Every weekend, she made the four-hour drive to Cleveland to visit her husband. She would treat his dressings, talk to him, and lay her head next to his shoulder.

"I couldn't really put my head on his chest because of the LVAD," says Brenda. "It was bulky and constantly made this *whirr-whirr* sound."

Yet the devices did their jobs as bridge therapies while Dan waited for a donor heart. The surgeons removed the RVAD within a few weeks. In early May, Dan was released to another hospital with a skilled nursing unit for physical therapy. He had spent months on bed rest with the assist devices, and he required lots of rehabilitation to be activated to the heart transplant list.

"I got stronger and better, but I still couldn't walk," says Dan. In June he was sent home, where a physical therapist visited him three days a week. "But I did the regimen every day on my own. I was determined that I was going to get stronger and walk and do things again." Only a week after returning home, Dan got "the call" telling him that a donor heart was available.

Receiving a donor heart

Dan answered the early morning phone call on June 21, 2005. "I thought, 'This is it! What do I do? I have to call everybody and get things together,'" he remembers. Dan and Brenda had planned on driving to the clinic, but that would take too long. We sent a Learjet to pick them up.

The transport team flew Dan to Cleveland Burke Lakefront Airport, drove him to the clinic, and delivered him to the staff who would prep Dan for transplant surgery. "It seemed like within an hour I was getting on the Learjet in Morgantown, West Virginia, then on the operating table," recalls Dan. "It was that fast. The clinic is so efficient, and everything fell into place."

Prior to the operation, Dan was allowed a few minutes to talk to his wife and family. Brenda remembers the brief conversation: "Dan said to me, 'I'll see you here or on the other side.' I said okay. But I was so confident in the staff at the clinic. Everything they had told me was going to happen so far had happened—good and bad."

Dan came through the four-hour surgery quite well, and the cardiac surgeon updated Brenda shortly after her husband's transplantation. Says Brenda, "He told me, 'I did the transplant, and Dan is doing well. He got a great heart.' That's all he said, and I never saw him again. It was like a visit from an angel."

While the thought of heart transplantation seems daunting to a healthy person, for Dan, who'd felt weak for years, then spent months on assist devices, the surgery was welcome. "The transplant was the easiest part of the whole ordeal," he says. "That evening, I talked to my family, my wife, and my stepkids." Then Dan began the six-week recovery process, including physical therapy and daily doses of antirejection drugs to help his body accept the donor heart.

A new lease on life

More than three weeks after surgery, Dan went home on a warm Saturday in July. "I immediately walked out on my back porch," he says. "I like to go out there and watch the birds. My wife couldn't get me to come back into the house." The surgery gave Dan a second chance at life, but it was still far from the active life he'd prized before his illness.

In his prime, Dan was a strapping man, standing more than six feet tall and weighing 200 pounds. He jogged, lifted weights, and did isometric exercises to strengthen and tone his muscles. Prior to the transplant, Dan had dwindled to 170 pounds and had a dangerously low ejection fraction of 8 percent.

Dan was eager to restore his health. The day after he returned home, he tried to stand a couple of times before getting in his wheelchair. He made it only halfway up. "The next morning, I tried to get up, and I did," he says. "I held onto the wall and walked into my stepson's room. I told him, 'I'm walking! I'm walking!' I called my wife at work to tell her the good news."

A physical therapist visited Dan regularly, helping him regain muscle strength through light aerobics, yoga, and other exercise. "I would take my walker and walk around the house one hundred ten times, which equals one mile," says Dan. "I was doing that twice a day."

It's now been more than a year since Dan's surgery. His ejection fraction hovers around 60 percent. He's back at work full time, and he walks nearly four miles almost every day in addition to lifting weights, riding a stationary bike, and doing yoga. He once again enjoys performing household tasks around his home in the woods: painting, mowing the lawn, trimming trees and bushes.

"Sometimes he gets so much energy," says Brenda. "We planted some hemlock trees in our side yard this spring.

He was going at it, and I was getting tired. He joked, 'You don't have a younger person's heart in you.'"

Dan still takes a host of medications, nearly 24 pills a day, including immunosuppressive drugs, vitamins and mineral supplements, a calcium channel blocker to reduce his heart's workload, and more. He makes periodic trips to the clinic for outpatient biopsies to examine his heart muscle and adjust medications if necessary. And he has to live with the knowledge that he's got only about a 20 percent chance of being alive in 20 years: the survival rate for heart transplant recipients is 90 percent at 1 year, 75 percent at 5 years, and 60 percent at 10 years.

But thanks to the donor heart, Dan feels a renewed sense of vitality and faith he hasn't had in more than a decade. "It's been a mind-boggling experience. I can't believe I went through all this," says Dan. "I take one day at a time, one step at a time. I don't blow up about things I might have before. It's not worth it. I have more harmony in my life now than ever."

Family Ties: Genetics and Heart Failure

If you can inherit your blue eyes or dark hair from your parents, can you also trace disorders, such as heart failure, to them? It's possible.

Genetic disorders or diseases are caused by the abnormal expression of one or more genes. It can range from an isolated mutation in a single gene to a significant chromosomal abnormality involving an entire set of chromosomes. There are approximately 4,000 genetic disorders, with new ones being discovered continually. One of the most common is cystic fibrosis.

Cardiomyopathy often has a genetic component. Ninety percent of cases of hypertrophic cardiomyopathy are familial, while genetic factors may be responsible for 30 percent to 50 percent of cases of dilated cardiomyopathy. Dan is one of those cases.

Genetic screening revealed that he had inherited Becker's muscular dystrophy from his mother, even though his brother and three sisters all tested negative for the chromosomal abnormality. Dan opted not to have children of his own (he has two stepchildren) for fear of passing on the disorder to his biological offspring.

Since the early 1990s, disease-causing mutations have been located in genes that encode heart muscle cells with the ability to contract and in proteins that make up a heart cell's structure. More than 20 mutations on 15 genes have been attributed to dilated cardiomyopathy and more than 200 mutations on 10 genes to hypertrophic cardiomyopathy. Most are the result of a single defective gene.

Other genetic traits that contribute to heart failure are considered *complex*: they are probably due to the effects of a number of genes in combination with lifestyle and environmental factors. Family members are often afflicted with the same complex disorders, but because there isn't a simple pattern of inheritance, it's hard to determine a person's risk of getting or passing on the disorder. Hypertension and heart disease are two examples of complex disorders.

Parents, siblings, and children of patients with hypertrophic cardiomyopathy or dilated cardiomyopathy from an unknown cause should undergo regular screenings with electrocardiograms and echocardiograms. You also may consider genetic testing and counseling to confirm or disprove inheritance and to receive information on passing the condition to another generation.

Genetic testing typically involves analyzing human DNA, RNA, chromosomes, proteins, or certain metabolites. A negative test often reassures family members that the heart disorder will not occur in that person and not be transmitted to future generations. A positive test confirms the diagnosis. Some men and women who test positive may never show symptoms of the disease, but they should be monitored carefully by a doctor.

Chapter 6

Beta-Blockers: Mike's Story

"I was determined to beat the diagnosis. I wasn't going to let it get me. I was going to fight this tooth and nail for my wife and two kids."
—**Mike, diagnosed with heart failure and placed on the transplant list in 2005, at age 42**

M ike is indeed a fighter. I met him in June 2005, a month after he was Life Flighted to Cleveland Clinic and admitted to the heart failure intensive care unit. His ejection fraction was a precariously low 8 percent, and he suffered arrhythmias.

Mike was placed on the transplant list and received aggressive medical therapy while waiting for a donor heart. But what's most dramatic about Mike's story isn't so much how he got on the transplant list; it's how he got *off* it.

Mike never received a new heart. He didn't need one; a combination of medications helped heal his damaged heart.

Mike's Story: From the Ski Slopes to the ICU

Mike was an active family man, spending his free time with his wife, Michelle, and their 12-year-old daughter and 10-year-old son. In March 2005, he tackled the toughest slopes in Vail, Colorado, while on a ski trip with his family. But just two weeks later, Mike could barely climb the stairs at Great American Ball Park to watch the Cincinnati Reds on Opening Day.

Flulike symptoms, including weakness, nausea, and diarrhea, persisted for two weeks, so Mike visited his family doctor, who admitted him to a local hospital with influenza and pneumonia. A routine chest X-ray revealed that Mike's heart was swollen, and physicians ordered an angiogram to check for any blocked coronary arteries.

"That's when my wife intervened and said, 'You guys aren't a heart hospital. What if something is wrong? What are you going to do?'" recalls Mike. When the doctors said they would transfer Mike to a heart care center if problems arose, he and Michelle opted to switch to Cincinnati's Christ Hospital prior to further testing.

Once there, Mike underwent an angiogram and echocardiogram. The angiogram indicated no signs of blockage or heart disease. But the echo was less reassuring. Mike's ejection fraction was between 10 percent and 15 percent. "They were throwing numbers at us left and right, but we didn't know what anything meant," says Mike. "I was only forty-two years old. I still thought I had the flu."

Uncertain why Mike was ill and his heart was deteriorating, the hospital started him on a variety of medications. These included antibiotics for pneumonia, beta-blockers for his heart, diuretics to reduce the swelling, and the statin drug Lipitor to lower his cholesterol. "They were pumping me intravenously with everything they could, trying to get my body to bounce back," he recalls.

Mike's vomiting continued, and he was unable to keep down any medications. Between the beginning of April and early May, he lost nearly 30 pounds from his 200-pound frame. "I was just dwindling away," he says.

Yet Mike was determined to be home from the hospital in time to celebrate Michelle's birthday in mid-May. He succeeded and was released two days ahead of schedule. But there was no celebration. "There was no way I could take her out," says Mike. "I never even got out of my bed or the La-Z-Boy."

When he began passing out and having arrhythmias, Mike was readmitted to the hospital several days later,.

Not that he remembers much about it. "My recollection of the month of May is zero," he says. "I was completely out of it, dead to the world. There's a whole month of my life that's gone."

While Mike was oblivious, the medical staff around him worked diligently to save his life. In an attempt to stabilize Mike, doctors tried new medications in the intensive care unit, but he had an adverse reaction. "They didn't think I was going to make it through the night," says Mike. "My EF had dropped from fifteen percent to below eight percent. I looked like death warmed over—like a ninety-year-old man in a forty-two-year-old body."

The heart failure specialists at Christ Hospital felt that they had exhausted their options. They pulled Michelle into the hall. "They said, 'The reason there are transplants in this world is for people like your husband,'" she remembers. "They said there was no alternative, and they were going to transfer Mike to a hospital that could do the transplant."

The physicians asked Michelle to share the news with Mike, and for the first time in this entire ordeal, she broke down. "I just couldn't tell my husband that," she says. So on May 23, with his parents, wife, one brother, and other family and friends surrounding him, Mike learned that he was going to be flown to Cleveland Clinic within the hour to begin evaluation for a heart transplant.

"Everyone was in tears," remembers Mike. "But I said, 'As bad as I feel, if that's what they have to do to make me better, then let's do it.'"

The fight of his life

Turbulent weather made the flight to Cleveland a choppy one, and Mike passed out midway through the journey. He made it to the heart failure intensive care unit, where he spent the next two weeks fighting for his life.

Mike received a Hickman catheter for medication, including the PDE inhibitor milrinone to improve his biventricular function and increase blood circulation. In addition, doctors inserted a pulmonary artery catheter to monitor his heart's performance. "I had so many tubes coming out of me that I looked like Frankenstein," he jokes.

Ten days after landing in the ICU, Mike stabilized and was coherent. The clinic began evaluating him for a heart transplant, when Mike suffered another setback. Doctors discovered a pulmonary embolism in his lungs, a mitigating factor that prevented Mike from going on the organ transplant list. He was given the blood thinner heparin to help resolve the blood clot.

Mike seemed caught in a web of medical conflicts: he couldn't receive a transplant because of the blood clot, and the medication prescribed to relieve the clot prevented him from receiving a pacemaker and defibrillator to thwart his arrhythmia. The doctors decided to take Mike off heparin for a few days to implant the potentially life-saving devices.

Meanwhile, Mike had insisted that his wife and children return to Cincinnati. The kids needed to finish the school year, and Michelle had to work. It was a scary, lonely time for him. "There were many nights, even before they left, that I'd send everyone out of the room and cry. Why me? What did I do?" he remembers.

Doctors implanted a pacemaker and defibrillator in early June; then Mike resumed the intravenous heparin to treat the clot. He set a goal: to be released in time to serve as a groomsman in a friend's wedding on June 10. After promising to take it easy, continue taking milrinone through his Hickman catheter, and line up a visiting nurse, Mike was granted his wish.

At that point, there wasn't much we could do at the clinic until the pulmonary embolism resolved itself, which could take several weeks. Although Mike was released from the hospital, he remained a high-risk patient reliant on medication to sustain his heart function. The defibrillator helped protect him from dying suddenly of arrhythmia, but he still had a 90 percent chance of dying within the next few months.

Mike's elation at being able to attend the wedding faded quickly. On the four-hour ride home with his wife and friend, he felt terrible. "It was probably the scariest drive of my life," he recalls. "I literally thought I was going to die. I had kept a good attitude through all this, but I didn't really think I was going to make it. I thought they were letting me go home to die."

Mike muddled through the wedding and rested at home for several days. Then one night, he decided to take Michelle and his kids to a little tavern for a bite to eat. Partway through the meal, Mike felt hot and woozy. He walked out to the parking lot to get some air and passed out in Michelle's arms. She laid him down in their truck and called an ambulance.

Three days later, Mike was readmitted to Cleveland Clinic and underwent numerous tests. He expected to fly home afterward. Instead he was moved to the hospital's transplant unit. The embolism was gone, and we anticipated that Mike would receive a donor heart within the week.

The waiting game

A few weeks passed, and still no heart became available. In the meantime, Mike continued taking milrinone, beta-blockers, and other medications. And he developed some habits that helped him remain upbeat.

First, Mike ditched the hospital gown. "I never dressed like I was in the hospital," he explains. "I put on shorts and T-shirts." He placed his portable heart monitor in the shirt pocket, with a hole cut out of the back to accommodate the wires leading to his chest. Second, Mike socialized with other transplant patients.

"I walked everyday on the treadmill next to a guy with an LVAD," he says. "I met a girl across the hall with cystic fibrosis who'd had a double lung transplant. We had coffee every day." He also gathered people for impromptu movie nights in the lounge at the end of the hall. His wife and kids would bring a movie, and they'd go room to room, telling patients about the flick. Together they'd watch the video and eat popcorn approved by a hospital dietitian.

"My kids loved sitting and watching a movie with their dad," says Mike. "I did whatever it took just to be with them." He often went outside with his IV bag hung on a pole with wheels—his "dance partner," he called it—to toss around a football with his son.

The nurses began to notice that Mike looked and seemed to feel much better than the average patient awaiting a transplant. I agreed and started to challenge the notion that transplantation was Mike's best option. So I had a candid conversation with him. I asked Mike whether he was willing to withdraw the milrinone, increase his beta-blockers, and see how his heart responded. He was game.

Mike realized there was a chance that at any time, he could crash, and his health would go downhill. But he said, "Let's go for it!" Day by day, I withdrew medications and told the transplant service to hold off providing a heart. Mike felt tired but good. By the end of July, his swollen heart had begun to shrink, and he was released. He was placed on the inactive transplant list, so we could continue to monitor him for several months.

Heart on the mend

I believe the primary reason for Mike's recovery was his body's response to the increased dosage of beta-blockers. While Mike, too, credits medicine and exercise, he thinks he was aided by the unconditional love and support of his family. "That's what pulled me through," he says. "I've got these two kids and my wife, and I had to get it together."

His kids still keep Mike on track today. If he tries to stray from his low-sodium diet, one of them will scold, "Daddy, you can't eat that!" Mike walks a mile or so each day and returns to the clinic regularly for checkups. His heart has nearly returned to its normal size, and his ejection fraction is between 40 percent and 45 percent.

We're still unsure what caused the heart failure, although our best guess is it was a virus. And I can't guarantee Mike that he won't relapse and have to go back on the transplant list. But right now, with all the data we have, Mike's prognosis is better than somebody who received a heart transplant. In fact, his five-year mortality rate is practically that of an average man his age.

Mike lives with gusto now, remaining particularly passionate about his hometown sports teams. By the fall of 2006, Mike was eagerly climbing the stairs at Paul Brown Stadium to watch his beloved Bengals from the seats he's had as a season-ticket holder for 12 years. Says Mike with a chuckle, "It's amazing to me what's happened in a year."

Caregivers Need Care, Too

Mike's wife, Michelle, and his two children were—and still are—his source of strength. But being there for a spouse or other family member with heart failure can be difficult.

Although Michelle remained strong in front of Mike, she admits that she often broke down when she left his bedside at the hospital. Her mind raced at night, and she couldn't sleep. So Michelle took sleeping pills for a while. But she also found support talking to other families with loved ones at the clinic.

As a caregiver, you'll probably help your family member navigate his or her condition, change diet and lifestyle, deal with mood swings, handle insurance and other financial issues, and much more. Here's some advice for you:

Acknowledge your feelings. You may get so wrapped up in dealing with the ailing person that you suppress your emotions. Are you afraid the patient might die? Do you feel responsible because you didn't help the person change bad habits long ago? Are you overwhelmed taking care of the patient and your children at the same time? These are all normal reactions. Make sure you share your thoughts with the patient, family members, friends, counselors, or others who can help. Your physician or hospital may be able to recommend a caregivers' support group.

Turn to other family members or friends for help. Being the sole caregiver for a person with heart failure can be overwhelming. Try to line up other people, whether family members or good friends, to drive the patient to and from doctor's appointments, pick up medication at the pharmacist, prepare nutritious meals for the rest of the family on days when the patient has procedures or tests, or provide other assistance.

Educate yourself about heart failure. Reading this book is certainly a great first step! The more you understand the condition, the more likely you are to feel in control and better able to help the patient. Keep a list of any questions you have about your loved one so that you can

On the Web: Support for Caregivers

A number of organizations provide support and advice to caregivers. Consider contacting these:

Heartmates
heartmates.com, (612) 558-3331

The Mended Hearts
mendedhearts.org, 888-432-7899/(214) 360-6149

National Caregivers Library
caregiverslibrary.org, (804) 327-1112

National Family Caregivers Association
nfcacares.org, 800-896-3650/(301) 942-6430

Well Spouse Association
wellspouse.org, 800-838-0879/(732) 577-8899

ask doctors or nurses at each appointment. In addition, learn about healthy diets for heart failure patients and other lifestyle changes. See Chapter 12: Living with Heart Failure for specific ideas.

Understand the patient's insurance policy. While your main concern is undoubtedly the health of the person with heart failure, the unfortunate reality is that insurance and other financial issues will come into play. Make sure that you have a copy of the insurance policy. You should know what the plan covers, whether treatments need to be precertified, how to submit claims, and other requirements. In addition, if the patient was the primary earner in the household, check with his or her employer about disability insurance, if necessary.

Take some time off. Set aside time for yourself when you can see a movie, meet a friend for lunch, take a long walk—whatever rejuvenates you. Caregivers often get burned out assisting the patient. Remember: your physical, mental, and emotional health are equally important, so make time for yourself.

Chapter 7

Life-Support Therapy: Kim's Story

"I cried myself to sleep many nights. When you are thirty years old, your ejection fraction should be higher than your age. I had just discovered what I wanted to do with my life in the last couple of years. Not knowing if I could ever do it again was devastating."
—Kim, diagnosed with heart failure in 2006, at age 30

In her late 20s, Kim finally found a career where she thrived: nursing. She worked with trauma patients in the intensive care unit at a hospital in Toledo, Ohio. It was during one of her shifts that Kim realized that her recent sluggishness and inability to catch her breath was caused by more than a bad cold.

An ECG revealed her heart rate was above 150 beats per minute, about twice the normal rate. In addition, Kim's blood pressure was quite low. Within a couple of weeks, her condition went downhill rapidly. She was diagnosed with *lymphocytic myocarditis,* which is inflammation of the heart muscle.

When I met Kim in early July 2006, she was in cardiogenic shock: her heart was so damaged that it couldn't pump enough blood to the rest of the body. The medical team here at Cleveland Clinic debated her options. Should we replace her heart with an artificial one? Did she have a chance at recovery?

With our guidance, Kim made some difficult choices regarding treatment. Ultimately she survived, and the story she tells is a compelling one.

Kim's Story: A Lingering Cold

Kim's problems began with a terrible cold. In late May 2006, she traveled to Cleveland with her sister for a fun weekend, starting with a Pearl Jam concert that Friday evening. But while the rock band belted out its song

"Comatose" during an encore, Kim felt, well, nearly comatose. She was congested and her head ached.

Not willing to give up on the weekend, Kim went with her sister to an Indians baseball game the next day. It was a dreary, bone-chilling day, and by the sixth inning, Kim had had enough. "I felt miserable," she recalls. "I was blowing my nose in napkins the whole game, so I told my sister we needed to leave so I could get some cold medicine." They stopped at a gas station for medicine, then drove back to Toledo.

At home, Kim loaded up on over-the-counter medication and struggled through a couple of night shifts at the hospital. Then she took off a few days, hoping that rest would cure her cold. After several weeks, her symptoms tapered off, and Kim thought she was on the mend. During another weekend away with her sister, Kim realized that she was mistaken.

The two drove north to Detroit to see the popular musical *Wicked*. They had front-row balcony seats. "We started to climb the stairs. During the first flight, I was winded," says Kim. "Thankfully, there was a crowd of people in front of us, so we were moving slowly. But by the first landing, I was gasping for air. I could feel my heart pounding."

By the time Kim made it to her seat, she was lightheaded. "I just didn't feel right," she says. "I thought, 'This is not normal with as much as I exercise.'" Two years prior, Kim weighed 250 pounds. She had lost more than 100 pounds through a low-carb diet and aerobic exercise, including cycling classes and running. Now a fit five-foot-six, the 30-year-old woman knew something was wrong.

She assumed that her cold had progressed to pneumonia or bronchitis and decided to call the doctor on Monday. But first she had to make it through her Sunday night shift at the hospital.

A diagnosis of cardiomyopathy

"When I walked to the department from the parking garage, I felt tired and sluggish," says Kim. "As the night wore on, I couldn't even walk to the bathroom without getting winded."

Partway through Kim's shift, the charge nurse gave her background information on a seriously ill patient. Kim joked that she might "code"—go into cardiac arrest—before the patient. The charge nurse questioned Kim about her symptoms, then insisted on performing an ECG and measuring her blood pressure. Kim's heart rate was a dangerously high 150 beats per minute, and her blood pressure was only 93/63.

Unwilling to be admitted at the hospital where she worked, Kim drove to the emergency room at another medical center. Doctors there administered another ECG, gave medicine to lower Kim's heart rate, and admitted her for 24-hour observation until she could be seen by her primary care doctor. "I did not want to stay in that hospital overnight," Kim recalls. "Little did I know I was going to be in the hospital for thirty-seven days."

The next morning, Kim's doctor visited and called for a cardiology consultation. He ordered basic blood tests and checked Kim's cardiac enzymes for signs of a heart attack.

A chest X-ray revealed that her lungs were clear, thereby ruling out pneumonia. Next the cardiologist called for an echocardiogram. "I still thought, 'I'm thirty years old. I'm fine. There's nothing wrong. He's just covering his bases,'" remembers Kim.

That evening, while she was chatting with her visiting sister and grandmother, the cardiologist entered her hospital room and asked to speak to Kim alone. "He sat on the edge of the bed and told me he had looked at the results of the echocardiogram and had some bad news," she says. "I had an EF of fifteen percent to twenty percent and serious cardiomyopathy. I'm a nurse. I knew what that meant. I started bawling."

The cardiologist suspected that the cause of her cardiomyopathy was viral, perhaps picked up during Kim's cold. The following morning, Kim underwent catheterization, and the doctors ruled out any blockages. They began treating Kim with a variety of medications, primarily beta-blockers, ACE inhibitors, and digoxin. She reacted poorly. "They all dropped my blood pressure and couldn't help my heart rate," Kim recalls.

The doctors tweaked the medication, but in the meantime, Kim began experiencing upper gastric problems and back pain. She was retaining fluid in her liver. After a week and a half of treatment with no progress, Kim was moved to the hospital where she worked. When a bedside echo revealed a clot in her right ventricle, Kim was transferred again, this time to Cleveland Clinic.

Kept alive by a machine

On July 3, Kim was admitted to the heart failure intensive care unit. Her heart was severely weakened and enlarged, unable to pump sufficient blood to her kidneys, lungs, and other organs. She also suffered from life-threatening arrhythmias.

Another echocardiogram confirmed a blood clot in Kim's heart. We inserted a catheter in a vein in her neck, snaked it to the right side of her heart, and began to monitor her cardiac function and adjust medications. A blood thinner, heparin, was started intravenously to treat the clot. Two days later, it was gone. Kim was taken off heparin, and we prepared her for a cardiac biopsy to assess her condition further.

The biopsy, which took approximately two hours, revealed lymphocytic myocarditis. It is extremely serious. Some patients become so sick they would die without an assist device to take over for the diseased heart. Other patients, however—even those who are very ill—have the capacity to recover. We hoped that Kim was one of them.

Unfortunately, oftentimes we can't tell which patients will recover, so we are very reluctant to replace their hearts until we've observed them for at least a few weeks or months. Most of the time, we simply don't know what causes myocarditis. We know that many common respiratory and flu viruses can cause the heart to become inflamed. In rare cases, some medications also can cause a drug-related myocarditis. There's no proven treatment beyond standard medications and therapies for heart failure. However, it may take at least three to six months to discover whether the heart will heal and recover.

In Kim's case, the cardiac surgeon and I considered options ranging from an artificial heart (which would be permanent) to assist devices (which can be temporary and are removed once the heart has recovered). While we pondered a course of action, Kim began to understand the gravity of her situation. "Before I even left the catheterization lab where they performed the biopsy, they had members from the transplant team in the room," she says. "They were introducing them to me."

Kim returned to her hospital room, where doctors inserted an intra-aortic balloon pump through a blood vessel in her groin and into the aorta to provide temporary assistance to the heart. The balloon pump is often used as a first step to see whether we can stabilize a patient. Unfortunately, it didn't help enough to make a difference for Kim.

Soon after, a cardiothoracic team recommended that she be put on an *ECMO* machine. ECMO, short for *extracorporeal membrane oxygenation,* is a life-support therapy in which a patient's blood is withdrawn from a large vein and passed through a pump into an artificial lung that oxygenates the blood and removes carbon dioxide. Then the blood is returned to the body. ECMO can provide temporary support for the right and left sides of the heart and the lungs.

Kim agreed to the procedure and was taken into surgery immediately. "I learned later that my EF at the time of the ECMO was only five percent, and I was a few hours from death," says Kim. "Thinking back, it did seem odd that they would do the surgery at night and not wait until the next morning."

ECMO is reserved for only the sickest patients at the clinic. Approximately 1 out of 5 who require ECMO don't survive. The odds were not in Kim's favor.

Twelve hours after the surgery commenced, she woke up in the intensive care unit on a ventilator. She grabbed a pad of paper and wrote a note to the nurses asking to have the air tube taken out. When the surgeons realized that she was alert and stable, they removed the ventilator.

The entire time that Kim was on ECMO, she had to lie flat on her back. When eating, she had to reach out without being able to see the food on her bedside tray; for upper body exercise, the young woman would lift small bags of saline, like weights. "I am not a person who sits still or watches TV," she says. "Even though I was weak and on ECMO, I hated lying around in the hospital."

Five days later, the heart surgeon and I discussed removing the ECMO machine and seeing how Kim would recover. We returned her to surgery to take out the machine and repair a blood vessel that had ruptured and caused a hematoma—a mass of clotted blood beneath the skin—at the site of the ECMO. Afterward, an echo showed that her EF had increased to 30 percent. Her blood pressure remained low, however, so Kim stayed in the ICU for a week or so more while we adjusted her medications.

A steady recovery

By the end of July, Kim was ready to be released from the hospital. Her EF remained around 25 percent, but her condition had improved enough that we felt she could manage her heart failure with medication.

The news about her discharge was extra special for Kim: it was July 26, her sister's birthday. Throughout the past couple of months, her sister had remained her biggest supporter. "I called her in Toledo to tell her I was coming home," Kim remembers. "She said, 'That's the best birthday present you could give me.'"

One of the first things Kim did when she got home was drive her new car, which she'd bought shortly before getting sick. She remained tired and slept a lot the first week. The following week, Kim returned to the gym and started walking slowly on the treadmill. "As hard as it was, I got myself up and started exercising," she says. "I went from feeling like I'd never be active again to gradually picking up my old life."

Her old life, but with a few key changes. Kim continues to take a number of medications, including beta-blockers, ACE inhibitors, diuretics, and mineral supplements. When she exercises, she wears a monitor to check her heart rate. Kim also eats more fruits and vegetables and watches her sodium and fluid intake. "I used to love French fries with salt, and I haven't had them since my discharge," she says. "It's just not worth the risk."

The memory of that summer spent fighting for her life rather than frolicking in the sun remains fresh in Kim's mind. "It's the scariest thing I've ever gone through," she says, taking a deep breath to choke back the tears. "Even though doctors tell you there's a chance you'll make it, you don't believe them."

In the fall, Kim visited her cardiologist in Toledo. He had good news: her EF had increased to 55 percent.

Nevertheless, the future is uncertain. It is possible that Kim may require additional therapies at some point, and she will remain on medications for the rest of her life. She'll also need to see a cardiologist regularly, and she understands that if her heart failure symptoms return, she should alert her doctor at once. But for now, the news is good indeed. Kim is one of the lucky ones who recovered.

Heart Failure and Women

When most people think of patients with cardiovascular disease, they conjure up images of overweight, middle-aged, or elderly men. But that's an inaccurate stereotype. According to the Cleveland Clinic Heart and Vascular Institute, cardiovascular disease is the number one killer of women over the age of 25 in the United States, regardless of race or ethnicity. In fact, the American Heart Association puts the number of American women affected by heart failure at approximately 2.6 million. As with other medical conditions, the causes, symptoms, and prognosis of heart failure in women may differ from those in men:

- Women tend to develop congestive heart failure at an older age than men.
- Women develop diastolic heart failure more often than men and more frequently than systolic heart failure. (Diastolic heart failure occurs when the heart pumps normally but the ventricles become stiff and

Pregnancy and Heart Failure

Cardiac diseases complicate 1 to 4 percent of pregnancies in women without preexisting cardiac abnormalities. Women who already have cardiomyopathy or heart failure and are contemplating pregnancy should carefully seek advice about their risks from their cardiologist and OBGYN. They should discuss contraception and maternal and fetal risks of pregnancy, some of which may be long-term or even life threatening.

On the Web: Women and the Heart

For more information on heart failure and women, try these Web sites:

HeartHealthyWomen.org
hearthealthywomen.org, (212) 851-9300

The National Coalition for Women with Heart Disease
womenheart.org, 877-771-0030/(202) 728-7199

The National Women's Health Information Center
4women.gov, 800-994-9662

The Cleveland Clinic–Pregnancy and Heart Disease Information
clevelandclinicmeded.com/medicalpubs/ diseasemanagement/cardiology/pregnancy-and- heart-disease/

don't relax properly, causing pressure to rise in the heart and lungs. In systolic heart failure, a weak heart can't contract with enough force, thereby preventing the body from receiving enough blood.)

- Women with heart failure are more likely than men to have high blood pressure, valvular disease, and diabetes mellitus and less likely to have congestive heart failure resulting from prior heart attacks.

- Although rare, woman can experience *peripartum cardiomyopathy*. This type of heart failure develops within the last month of pregnancy or within five months after delivery and occurs without an identifiable cause.

- While the symptoms of heart failure are the same among both sexes, women tend to experience more shortness of breath and more difficulty exercising than men. They also have swelling around their ankles more frequently than men.

- In general, women survive heart failure longer than men with the condition.

Chapter 8

Dor Procedure: Joe's Story

"When the doctors explained the operation to me, I said, 'Let's go for it!' What did I have to lose? If I went home, I'd die."
— Joe, heart attack survivor who underwent the Dor procedure in 1997, at age 67

Joe was one of the first patients to undergo the Dor procedure at Cleveland Clinic. Three and a half years earlier, he had suffered a heart attack that left his heart weakened and enlarged. When I met Joe in 1997, I thought he was headed toward a heart transplant. But we suggested the Dor procedure—a revolutionary course of action at the time—to see whether we could stabilize his condition and delay the transplant.

Joe agreed. "From the time I had my heart attack until my surgery in Cleveland, I was in and out of the hospital seventeen times, all for heart problems," he recalls. The husband and father of two was willing to try anything to combat his congestive heart failure.

What generally happens after a heart attack is that the heart gets increasingly larger, often to the point where nothing can be done. The goal of the Dor procedure is to reconstruct the heart, stop it from dilating, and avoid a transplant. Joe's operation was a success.

Asked about his heart today, Joe says simply, "It's still pumping!" That's an achievement, considering the strain it's been under since June 30, 1994.

Joe's Story: A Celebration Cut Short by a Heart Attack

On that muggy summer evening, Joe headed out of the aluminum plant where he was a supervisor. He hitched a ride with a couple of coworkers to a retirement party for another employee. An hour later, they arrived at a VFW hall.

"The place was packed with friends and people from work," Joe recalls. He drank a few beers and danced—even taking a spin on the floor with the retiree while onlookers hooted at the two men. It was a fun party, until Joe began to feel ill.

"I started sweating because it was hot, so I went outside with a beer and lit up a cigarette," he says. Shortly after, he threw up in a dumpster outside the hall. When his left arm started to ache, Joe suspected that something was really wrong, so he asked two friends to drive him back to his car at the plant.

"They wanted to take me to the hospital," says Joe. "I said, 'You're not taking me nowhere!'" He stubbornly drove home, a 90-mile trip on two-lane roads and the highway. "By the time I got home, the pain in my arm and chest was so bad. I know I should've stopped along the way at a hospital," he says. "But I thought, 'If I'm going to die, I want to see my wife and daughter first.'"

When Joe pulled into the driveway of his secluded West Virginia home, his daughter was outside chatting with a friend. "I opened the car door and hollered out to her, 'I'm having a heart attack. Call an ambulance!'" The paramedics rushed Joe to the local emergency room, where doctors confirmed Joe's self-diagnosis.

But he doesn't remember much from the ER. By the time he arrived there, Joe was unconscious, his breathing was shallow, and he had dangerously low blood pressure. He was in cardiac arrest, so doctors injected epinephrine into his heart to restart the organ. "I don't remember anything after that—not a damn thing," says Joe.

Joe regained consciousness the next day, when his family doctor visited him in the hospital. Because Joe remained unstable, the physician wanted to transfer him to a larger hospital in Charleston. Despite the gravity of the situation, Joe remained under the illusion that he could go home. "I told the doctor I had to go to work," he remembers. "We were shorthanded; one guy was out sick, and one was on vacation. I said I had to be there."

The doctor refused, insisting that Joe get further treatment in Charleston. Joe begrudgingly consented. The extent of his condition finally dawned on him when he went outside for transport to the bigger hospital. "I said, 'Which ambulance are we going on?' The doctor said, 'You're not.' And he pointed to a helicopter."

Joe remembers bits and pieces of the helicopter ride. He recalls looking down at the Kanawha River that meanders through the valleys and mountains surrounding West Virginia's capital. He also remembers landing on the hospital roof and a sea of white-clad people swarming the helicopter. After that, he lost consciousness until July 3.

"They told my wife that any relatives who wanted to see me should get there right away because I wasn't going to make it." Joe's son flew home from Hawaii, where he attended college. But Joe survived. He spent 14 days in the hospital before he was released with instructions to stay away from work until the new year. Instead Joe returned to the aluminum plant in September. "That was a big mistake," he admits.

Heart problems persist

Initially, Joe worked days. Then he went back to rotating shifts, as he had done before the heart attack. While driving to work for one midnight shift, he started experiencing chest pain again. For the next three years, he battled chest discomfort, arrhythmia, and shortness of breath, yet he continued to work. He had two stents inserted to keep his coronary arteries open.

By 1997, Joe was frustrated with his persistent symptoms and trips to the hospital. During one particularly bad night at work in August, his arrhythmia kicked up a storm and set off an all-too-familiar chain of events: Joe was once again rushed by ambulance to the hospital, was transported by helicopter to Charleston, and spent a week in the hospital.

Afterward, Joe confronted his family physician, who told the patient there was little else he could do for him. Joe refused to accept defeat. "Are you telling me to go home and die?" he asked the doctor. "I'm not going to die. You find me someone, somewhere, to get me better." A week later, a nurse called and suggested that Joe visit me at Cleveland Clinic.

That fall, Joe underwent a battery of tests at the clinic. In addition to congestive heart failure, he had an aneurysm: a big area on his heart had ballooned out, and the blood flowed around it. The cardiac surgeon and I considered options, including a heart transplant. But we decided a combination Dor procedure and bypass surgery might delay the need for transplantation. Joe agreed, despite the very real risk that he might not survive the innovative procedure.

Less than a week before Christmas, Joe was wheeled into the operating room. The surgeon performed a double bypass, grafting new blood vessels to circumvent two blocked arteries and restore normal blood flow to Joe's heart. During the

Dor procedure, the surgeon reconstructed the left ventricle by placing a row of circular stitches around the dead tissue to cut it off from the healthy tissue and shrink the heart.

"Two days after the surgery, I woke up with tubes down my throat," Joe recalls. When the hospital staff removed the tubes, Joe's onslaught of questions reassured them that he was feeling okay. "I asked them what day it was, and they said it was Sunday," recalls Joe. "Then I asked what time it was, and they said 1 P.M. So I asked whether I could watch football on TV."

Joe recovered nicely after the operation and was sent home in time for Christmas. Although he still was in pain from the major surgery, Joe was optimistic that his heart problems were behind him. That optimism was short lived.

Two days into the new year, Joe's wife was forced to call the ambulance yet again. "I went upstairs to get my slippers on, bent down in front of the closet, and the room went dark," remembers Joe. "I passed out and fell down."

Joe was admitted to the hospital in Charleston. His heart was racing, so he was given medication to slow it down. The medicine was ineffective. In February Joe received a defibrillator. But that still didn't end his medical turmoil.

Several times during the spring of 1998, Joe's defibrillator went off, shocking his heart back into rhythm. One time it happened while Joe was in the hospital overnight for tests; he was in the bathroom brushing his teeth. "All of a sudden, I saw silver in my eyes. It looked like aluminum foil. And I heard humming in my ears," says Joe. "I grabbed the sink because I knew I was going to go down. I hit the shower curtain, and thank God a nurse came in."

Technicians confirmed that Joe's defibrillator had gone off several times. His medication was adjusted, and since then the defibrillator has remained inactive. Aside from a bout of pneumonia in 1999, Joe's health has remained stable.

A new lifestyle

After his five-year medical saga, Joe is glad to have his life back—although it's very different from the one he led before his heart attack. Like many patients with heart failure, Joe is on a daily regimen of pills, including cholesterol-lowering medication, a diuretic, a blood thinner, an angiotensin II receptor blocker, and mineral supplements. He rarely drinks alcohol, watches his diet, and walks his dogs several times a day for exercise.

Perhaps the biggest change is that Joe, once a workaholic, has retired. "I had fifty people working for me at the plant," he says. "I was responsible for the quality of the work, the quantity we output, and my employees' safety." The stress, he contends, was too much. Joe hasn't worked at the plant in a decade. But he's not one to sit still, so he has taken over all the housecleaning duties at home.

Looking back, Joe reflects on how his ordeal transformed his mind-set as well as his activities. "In the beginning, when all this happened, I felt sorry for myself. I really did. I kept saying, 'Why me?' Then the doctor said it was my lifestyle." Joe chuckles and adds, "I had a damn good life-style before my heart attack. Then I realized that was stupid, and I stopped feeling sorry for myself. It happened, and you can't do anything about it. You can't go back."

More on the Dor Procedure

Since Joe's surgery in 1997, more than 250 similar procedures have been performed at Cleveland Clinic. The operation is named after Vincent Dor, a cardiac surgeon in Monte Carlo, Monaco, who has refined the procedure and written numerous scientific articles in medical journals. The operation is also known as *surgical anterior ventricular remodeling (SAVR), surgical ventricular restoration (SVR),* and sometimes simply *aneurysectomy.*

During the last ten years, we have learned that the Dor procedure can be performed safely with a mortality rate of under 5 percent. It appears to stabilize patients, thereby postponing the need for heart transplantation. A patient's quality of life improves, and fewer hospitalizations are necessary. However, proving the efficacy and safety of the Dor procedure will require a large, well-designed clinical trial. In fact, a worldwide study is currently under way at 90 leading medical centers to provide definitive answers to these important questions.

The trial, called STICH (Surgical Treatments for Ischemic Heart Failure), hopes to determine the optimal therapy for people with heart failure brought about by coronary artery disease. Doctors will be comparing the outcomes from (1) medication alone, (2) medication plus coronary artery bypass surgery, and (3) medication, CABG, and surgical ventricular restoration. We hope to learn the results in the next two or three years. (More information is available online at *stichtrial.org*.) For now, Cleveland Clinic and many other hospitals around the world continue to perform the Dor procedure in patients they think are most likely to benefit. Hopefully, each patient will fare as well as Joe.

When to Seek Medical Attention

In the span of a decade, Joe was in and out of the hospital on close to 20 occasions and taken there by ambulance a handful of times. Nobody wants to spend that much time in a medical facility. But unexpected visits between your regular doctor appointments may be necessary.

Call your physician if you experience any of the symptoms listed here:

- Unexplained weight gain (more than two pounds in a day or five pounds in a week)
- Swelling in your ankles, feet, legs, or abdomen that worsens
- Shortness of breath that becomes worse or occurs more frequently; waking up short of breath
- A bloated feeling in your stomach with a loss of appetite or nausea
- Extreme fatigue or the inability to complete daily activities

- A respiratory infection or cough that becomes worse
- A heart rate of 120 beats per minute or more
- A new, irregular heartbeat
- Chest pain or discomfort during activity that is relieved with rest
- Difficulty breathing during regular activities or at rest
- Changes in your sleep, including insomnia or excessive sleep
- Decreased urination
- Restlessness or confusion
- Constant dizziness or lightheadedness
- A poor appetite or nausea

Call 911 or go to the emergency room if you experience any of the following:

- New chest pain or discomfort that is severe or unexpected and is accompanied by shortness of breath, sweating, nausea, or weakness
- A heart rate of 120 to 150 beats per minute, accompanied by shortness of breath
- Shortness of breath that can't be relieved by rest
- Sudden weakness or paralysis in your arms or legs
- A sudden, severe headache
- A fainting spell with loss of consciousness

Chapter 9

Heart Transplant: Jennifer's Story

"People always ask, 'What did you think when the doctors said you needed a heart transplant?' Maybe I'm weird, but I just thought, 'Okay, if that's what we have to do, then let's do it.'"
— Jennifer, recipient of a heart transplant in 2004, at age 29

Jennifer has been a go-getter all her life: She played piano competitively for 15 years. She danced ballet *en pointe*—on the tips of her toes—which requires considerable strength and skill. Before she was 30, she had completed an accelerated medical school program through Louisiana State University and landed a fellowship in pediatric cardiology. It's no surprise, then, that when a rare inflammatory disease suddenly attacked Jennifer's heart, she fought back with determination and optimism.

Within a matter of weeks during the summer of 2004, Jennifer plummeted from a hard-working doctor making rounds to a bedridden patient awaiting a heart transplant. She was extremely weak, in a lot of pain, and kept alive only with a biventricular assist device. Yet Jennifer remained hopeful and demonstrated remarkable fortitude.

Jennifer's Story: A Mysterious Condition Strikes Fast

Exhausted. Truly exhausted. That's how Jennifer felt the last week of August. But she wasn't surprised or concerned. The 29-year-old had spent the past couple months as a fellow at Cincinnati Children's Hospital Medical Center. Her normally busy schedule was even more hectic that week, as Jennifer picked up the workload of a colleague who was out of town for a funeral.

Jennifer had been on call five out of six days. "I was really tired at the end of that stretch, but that's par for the course for a cardiology fellow," she says. "But I also got short of breath walking up one flight of stairs to my office. That was odd."

A healthy young woman, Jennifer previously had no problems dancing the night away with friends. So why was she now weary climbing a dozen or so steps? On August 30, Jennifer made a fateful decision to find out. "On the way out of the hospital at 8:30 at night after all my calls, I went to the echo lab and did an ultrasound on myself," she recalls.

The results were disturbing: Jennifer discovered fluid around her heart. She called her attending physician to say that she'd be late for rounds the next morning. When Jennifer explained why, the doctor insisted she go to the emergency room.

"My thought was that it was a viral thing, because that's the most common explanation for fluid around the heart," says Jennifer. She felt confident that she would receive medication and be sent home.

Prior to going to the ER, Jennifer took two other steps. First she took her blood pressure at the recommendation of an adult cardiologist who was a friend of her boyfriend Chad, also a doctor. It was very low: around 80/50. Next she paged a friend who was an ultrasound technician to perform a complete echocardiogram. "It's so hard to echo yourself, and I wanted a recording of my echo to bring to the ER," says Jennifer.

Afterward, she headed to the emergency room. "I really started going downhill," Jennifer recalls. "My blood pressure dropped, my heart was out of rhythm, and I went into cardiac tamponade." In this emergency condition, the sac covering the heart fills with fluid, which prevents the ventricles from expanding fully and adequately pumping blood.

"Usually that happens over a fair amount of time," explains Jennifer. "But five or six hours after my initial echo, I was in tamponade and going to the catheterization lab. I don't remember much because I was completely out of it." Doctors inserted a catheter into Jennifer's heart to remove the fluid and relieve pressure. Then she was sent to the intensive care unit, where the staff treated her for viral myocarditis.

But Jennifer didn't respond. Her blood pressure remained low, her ejection fraction dipped to 30 percent, and she experienced life-threatening arrhythmias. A variety of experts, from infectious-disease specialists to pulmonologists, searched in vain to discover what was attacking Jennifer's heart.

"I was in the ICU for two days when they decided I needed to be transferred somewhere that could offer me a transplant," says Jennifer. On September 1, she was flown to Cleveland Clinic.

Kept alive with assist devices

Being a doctor was both a blessing and a curse for Jennifer during her ordeal. While she could knowledgably advocate on her own behalf, she sometimes knew too much. One of those times was on the flight to Cleveland. "Chad and I were the only doctors on the plane," recalls Jennifer. "I started having arrhythmias, and I remember one of the technicians showing me the irregular rhythms." Jennifer knew she was in bad shape.

"I started having a lot of chest discomfort," she says. "Basically, my heart was dying."

The plane landed, and an ambulance rushed Jennifer to the clinic, where she was admitted to the heart failure intensive care unit.

While Jennifer hovered near death, her family launched into action. Her brother, who was in medical residency in Atlanta, and her parents, who lived in Baton Rouge, Louisiana, had traveled to Cincinnati. They arrived the same day that Jennifer was brought to Cleveland. "My brother told me afterward that my dad, who teaches at LSU, asked whether he should come up to Cleveland," says Jennifer. "He asked whether the situation was really that bad, and my brother said, 'Yes!'"

Her brother was right: almost as soon as Jennifer arrived at the clinic, she went into cardiac arrest. "They were trying all kinds of stuff: an intra-aortic balloon pump to assist my heart and a pulmonary artery catheter to monitor my heart," Jennifer recounts. "Nothing really worked." Doctors then administered inotropic heart medication to help her heart muscles contract.

"I sat up, stared at Chad with a weird look, and had a seizure," says Jennifer. "I remember being scared. I could hear, but I couldn't move. I heard the nurses say, 'She's going into arrest!' Then I could feel the shock. I saw a blinding white light. It's indescribable." Using a defibrillator, doctors were able to restore Jennifer's heart rhythm—for the moment.

Jennifer was so unstable that one of my partners, Dr. Robert E. Hobbs, was called at 4:30 in the morning. He suspected that Jennifer had *giant cell myocarditis,* a rare disease that causes the body's immune system to attack the heart. Unless patients receive transplants or are supported with mechanical devices, death is almost certain.

Dr. Hobbs immediately assembled an emergency surgical team to implant a biventricular assist device. "My heart wasn't doing any kind of rhythm," recalls Jennifer. "Through shocking, the doctors bridged me enough to get to the operating room. I'm sure if it had taken much longer, I wouldn't even be alive today."

On September 2, Jennifer was hurried to surgery. Minutes before the procedure, she went into cardiac arrest and was revived, again. Jennifer then received two ventricular assist devices, one for each of her heart's lower chambers. Afterward, she was taken to the intensive care unit, where she remained unconscious for a day and a half. Soon after she woke up, Jennifer received a report from pathology confirming Dr. Hobbs's diagnosis of giant cell myocarditis. The condition, said to be idiopathic because we don't know its cause, is named for the presence of abnormal clumps of fused cells that originate from certain white blood cells. These giant cells then infiltrate and destroy cardiac tissue.

While the biventricular assist devices were doing the work for Jennifer's diseased heart, it wasn't a permanent solution. When I visited Jennifer at her bedside as she recovered from surgery, I explained that she had two options. One was to try immunosuppressive therapy. The other was to place her on the transplant list.

I was involved in clinical trials where we gave immuno-suppressant drugs to patients with giant cell myocarditis. The goal was to lower the body's immune response to bacteria, viruses, and other foreign agents, then work to reduce inflammation of the heart and improve its function. However, immunosuppressive therapy was generally beneficial to patients less critically ill than Jennifer.

My goal was to get her transplanted, then administer the immunosuppressants with the new heart. Jennifer agreed, and we placed her as a status 1A candidate for transplantation—the highest priority for those on organ waiting lists.

Waiting for a heart

Jennifer began the waiting game, with the humming sound of the heart pumps visible on her abdomen a constant reminder that her life hung in the balance. "I had tubes coming out of everywhere, and I couldn't really move," she says.

Through it all, Jennifer remained steadfast. "I wasn't stressed out the whole time I was waiting because I truly felt I would get a heart," she says. "In hindsight, I feel lucky because the waiting list is long."

Jennifer spent most of her time sleeping. Lots of friends flew to Cleveland to visit her. "But I was in and out of it," she says. "I know I didn't have good conversations." Most of her memories of this time concern simple things that people usually take for granted, like her daily sponge bath. "Nurses had to help me with everything," says Jennifer. "I was a modest person before, but once you go through that, you're not modest anymore."

Ten days after her biVAD surgery, Jennifer woke up on a Sunday morning. "I hadn't heard anything about a donor heart, and I was bummed," she remembers. The young doctor knew that hearts and other organs often become available during weekends, when accidents are more prevalent. "It's a bittersweet reality," says Jennifer.

That evening the transplant team told Jennifer a compatible heart was available. She was elated—and really scared for the first time. "Having open heart surgery twice in a week or so is hard on the body," she says. "Being a physician, I understood too much about transplantation. I know it's high risk." Between 5 percent and 7 percent of transplant patients don't survive more than 30 days after the surgery.

Jennifer's room buzzed with preparation for her operation. One member of the team helped soothe her nerves. "A cardiothoracic technician came in and held my hand all the way into the operating room until I fell asleep under anesthesia," she says.

The surgery began late in the evening on September 12. Six hours later, Jennifer had a new heart. A longtime friend who'd flown to Cleveland to support her says, "A mere twelve hours after her transplant, she was alert, talking, drinking fluids, and craving a cup of coffee and a Big Mac. She is truly an inspiration!"

The long road of rehab

Jennifer would need to call on her strong spirit throughout her arduous recovery. Many heart transplant patients are sick for so many years prior to surgery that they feel dramatically better afterward. Jennifer had the opposite experience: because her illness came on rapidly and severely damaged her heart within a couple weeks, she struggled postsurgery. "The rehab, for me, was difficult mentally because I was fine before," she admits.

Jennifer remained in the clinic for 18 days after surgery. She took oral immunosuppressive drugs and was treated with corticosteroids for early rejection. She was very weak. Each day, nurses would move her to a chair for 20 minutes. "I did not like being up. I was really dizzy," she recalls.

Jennifer had lost muscle mass lying in a bed for nearly two weeks prior to the transplantation. It was a challenge to get up and brush her teeth. She even had a bedside toilet because she couldn't walk the few steps to the bathroom. "When you're that sick, you have these small goals that make you happy," she says. "One of the best things was washing my hair, because I hadn't done it since I got sick."

In November, Jennifer was well enough to return to Cincinnati, where she moved in with Chad. Her mother also stayed with them while Jennifer regained her strength. There were setbacks in recovery: Jennifer was hospitalized once after Thanksgiving, when the medications upset her stomach. She takes approximately 40 pills a day, including antirejection drugs, mineral supplements, low-level steroids, and a bisphosphonate to combat bone loss from the steroids.

At times Jennifer was frustrated by the slow recovery. "Then I realized that it's okay to have days where I feel that life's unfair," she reflects.

At the end of November, Jennifer insisted that her mom return to Louisiana. "Her life centered around me for so long, I wanted her to go home," says Jennifer. "I wanted her to know that I'd be okay."

By Christmas Jennifer was walking two miles and lifting two-pound weights. "Watch out, Governor Schwarzenegger!" she teased. She visited friends, baked dozens of holiday cookies, and even played in the snow for a few minutes. The Southerner enjoyed her first white Christmas.

Still, adjusting to her new life—and new heart—was a gradual process. "It took me six months before I felt like the heart was mine," says Jennifer. "When I would go to sleep at night, I could hear it beating in my ears." She used to talk about the transplanted heart as a separate entity—someone else's heart. Over time, however, it became hers.

A second chance at life

In 2004 Jennifer was a dynamic young woman with limitless opportunities. Since the transplant, the most difficult transition has been accepting limitations.

When her childhood home was hit by Hurricane Katrina, she couldn't travel to Louisiana and help with the cleanup because the unsanitary conditions would compromise her health. She felt helpless. But the determined doctor found a way to lend a hand: Jennifer volunteered at a Red Cross evacuee clinic in Cincinnati, assessing patients with noninfectious issues and writing prescriptions.

She's had to alter her dream of working as a pediatric cardiologist, too. "That's been the hardest part," says Jennifer. "I couldn't do what I was trained to do. I couldn't be around sick people." But she hasn't abandoned pediatrics altogether. Jennifer moved back to Atlanta, where she now works in a hospital's well-baby nursery. "I've even diagnosed a couple of babies with cardiac problems," she says. "It's not what I was doing before, but the pace of it is good for now."

With more time on her hands and a renewed appreciation for life, Jennifer has cultivated relationships. "I was very, very busy before, to the point of not calling people back," she says. "Now I take more time, even if it's just to send a short email to a friend I haven't seen in a month or so."

And the most important relationship in her life has also blossomed: Chad and Jennifer are getting married this year. They will honeymoon in the South Pacific, then settle into the 100-year-old house they recently purchased. Jennifer knows the odds are slim that she'll grow old with Chad: the 20-year survival rate for heart transplant patients is approximately 20 percent, and a second transplant may be another challenge she will have to face someday. But she embraces life with gusto and encourages other heart failure patients to do the same.

"I tell people waiting for a transplant that it gets better. It may take awhile, but it gets better," says Jennifer. "If you're a transplant patient, you've been given the ultimate gift. It really is the gift of life."

The Fundamentals of Organ Donation

In August 2007, more than 2,600 patients in the United States were on the waiting list for heart transplants, according to the Organ Procurement and Transplantation Network (OPTN), which maintains the national patient waiting list. How did they get on the list? And what happens once they're listed?

The process of organ transplantation is regulated by the Health Services and Resources Administration of the U.S. Department of Health and Human Services, which contracts with the United Network for Organ Sharing (UNOS) to maintain a centralized computer network linking all organ procurement organizations and transplant centers. The network facilitates every organ transplant in the United States and is accessible 24 hours a day, 7 days a week.

After a patient is referred by a doctor, a transplant center evaluates the person's physical and mental health for possible transplant. As of August 2007, Cleveland Clinic was one of 135 heart transplant programs in the United States, according to UNOS. When patients are considered good candidates for transplantation, their medical profiles are added to the waiting list.

There are three main status categories for people on the waiting list:

- *Active patients* are those whose conditions are favorable for transplantation.
- *Inactive patients* have conditions that temporarily prevent transplant surgery, such as infections.

On the Web: Organ Donation and Transplantation

For more information on transplantation, visit one of these Web sites:

Heart Failure Society of America
hfsa.org, (651) 642-1633

International Society for Heart & Lung Transplantation
ishlt.org, (972) 490-9495

Organ Procurement and Transplantation Network
optn.org, 888-894-6361

United Network for Organ Sharing
unos.org, 888-894-6361

U.S. Department of Health and Human Services
organdonor.gov

- *Removal status* is for patients who have been taken off the list for any of several reasons. For instance, they may have died, recovered adequate organ function, received a transplant, or become too ill.

When an organ becomes available, a matching system generates a ranked list of potential recipients based on organ type, geographic area, genetic compatibility, the severity of the candidate's disease, and numerous other criteria. The organ is then offered to the transplant team of the first person on the list. If the patient is available and healthy enough to undergo surgery, lab tests are run to ensure the organ is a good match. Once a recipient is selected and the testing is done, then surgery is scheduled and the transplant takes place.

Donor hearts come from people who have been declared brain-dead and whose families consent to donating the organ. Typically, brain death occurs due to a head injury from a car accident, gunshot wound, or hemorrhage in the brain. It's an anonymous gift.

Chapter 10

Cardiac Resynchronization: Ambrose's Story

"I was hunting during small-game season in November 2004, running up and down mountains. I felt winded, but I didn't think too much of it. I just thought I was out of shape."

—Ambrose, diagnosed with heart failure in 2004

Ambrose was an average middle-aged man in the fall of 2004. He was married with three grown children. He worked in the engineering department of a powdered metal plant that makes gears and other parts for the automotive industry. He liked to golf in the summer and hunt in the winter.

Ambrose didn't adhere to a set exercise regimen, but he occasionally used a treadmill. He ate the standard American diet: lots of processed foods high in fat and low in fiber and complex carbohydrates. And he liked drinking a beer or two when he relaxed.

But his life changed dramatically late that year, when within a couple of weeks, he progressed from being winded to feeling as though he couldn't breathe. Ambrose's father had died of a heart arrhythmia at 71. His sister died of heart failure at 47. He knew his symptoms were serious.

By the time Ambrose entered my office in early 2005, his ejection fraction was 15 percent, his heart had enlarged to more than 7 centimeters, he looked terrible, and he had typical signs and symptoms of heart failure.

Ambrose's Story: The Ol' Family Diagnosis

On a weekend in November 2004, Ambrose was exactly where he loved to be: hunting in the mountains of northern Pennsylvania. But he wasn't having much fun tracking deer with his friends. "We were putting on a drive, and I told one of them, 'Wait for me at the top of the hill. I'll be a little slow,'" recalls Ambrose. "I could feel something was wrong, but I didn't know what."

Despite being hampered by shortness of breath that day, Ambrose made plans to hunt the following weekend with one of his sons. "The night before, I went to bed with all intentions of getting up in the morning to go hunting," he says. "But I couldn't sleep. I lay down, and I couldn't breathe. The only way I could breathe was if I sat up in a chair."

After a restless night in his recliner, Ambrose called his son on Saturday morning to cancel the hunting trip. "I told him, 'If I go hunting today, there's no way I'm coming back.'" While Ambrose felt a bit better, he was only able to doze on and off that weekend, having to remain upright.

Monday morning, Ambrose visited his family doctor, who ordered an electrocardiogram. The ECG revealed a *bundle branch block.* Bundle branches are fibers of specialized tissue that travel to the right and left ventricles, allowing electrical signals that control the heart's pumping to stimulate both chambers at the same time. This coordinated contraction of the ventricles is essential for optimal pumping of the blood to the body and lungs. When a bundle branch is blocked, one of the ventricles contracts just after the other one. Ambrose had left bundle branch block, which is seen in almost 30 percent of patients with heart failure.

His doctor suspected heart failure and asked Ambrose to return the following day for an echocardiogram and stress test. The echo showed an extremely low ejection fraction of 15 percent, and the stress test results were equally alarming. "I was on the treadmill for about fifteen seconds when the doctor said, 'That's enough!' and cut it off," says Ambrose.

The physician told him to consult a cardiologist, so he made an appointment with the same one who had treated his sister several years prior. "When I first heard my EF was fifteen percent, I started to think about my sister," says Ambrose. "When she was first diagnosed with heart failure, hers was thirty percent to thirty-five percent, and it kept decreasing. I thought if this happened to my sister and she went downhill that quickly, then, boy, am I in trouble!"

Ambrose had vivid memories of his sick sister, who died four years before his own diagnosis. He used to pick her up and bring her to one of his sons' high school basketball games. "She would get around and try to do as much as possible, but she couldn't go for very long," says Ambrose. "She got winded very quickly."

The cardiologist examined the test results and placed Ambrose on a beta-blocker, ACE inhibitor, and diuretic. Ambrose also followed the physician's orders to lower his salt and fluid intake and stop drinking beer. But throughout December, he got weaker and weaker. By the end of the month, he had lost nearly 25 pounds.

Ambrose opted for a second medical opinion. "I didn't have any problem with my cardiologist, but I'd read a lot about Cleveland Clinic," he says. "I thought if anything happens, I wanted to be there."

Fainting leads to cardiac resynchronization therapy

On January 3, 2005, Ambrose drove nearly four hours to the clinic for his first consultation. During the next three days, we ran several tests: I ordered an electrocardiogram, which showed a significant electrical conduction delay, and another echocardiogram, which indicated a 10 percent ejection fraction. Ambrose also underwent cardiac catheterization to confirm that he didn't have any blocked arteries and had not suffered a heart attack.

I explained to Ambrose that his heart failure was severe, and together we formulated a care plan that involved adjusting his medications and frequent monitoring. After scheduling a follow-up appointment in February, he returned home on January 5. "The next morning, we had a snowstorm," Ambrose recalls. "I was standing at the front door directing my two boys as they shoveled the snow, and I collapsed." His sons called an ambulance, and Ambrose was rushed to a local hospital. Doctors there could not find anything new amiss, so he was sent home that afternoon.

The following week, Ambrose felt so drained that he missed all but one day of work. Then Sunday in church, he passed out again. "The priest had finished the sermon and started the consecration at Mass. I felt weak and sat down," remembers Ambrose. "My wife asked if I was okay, and I said I'd be all right. Then I started seeing flashes and collapsed."

A nurse in the congregation rushed to Ambrose's side, laid him on the floor, and checked his vitals. She couldn't find a pulse. Just as the ambulance arrived, Ambrose came around. "The local hospital called the clinic this time, and they said, 'Get him out here!'" says Ambrose. Later that afternoon, an ambulance transported him to the clinic, where he was examined and monitored.

"I thought when I went to Cleveland that I was going to need a heart transplant," says Ambrose. "My sister was on the transplant list, and in my mind, that's what heart failure always deteriorates into." But recent medical developments had changed the outcome for many heart failure patients, even in the few years since his sister's death.

The following morning, I talked with Ambrose about his condition. Because of his fainting episodes, we altered our original plan of tracking his condition for nine months or so. I suggested cardiac resynchronization therapy (CRT), a relatively new treatment designed to relieve the symptoms of heart failure and improve coordination of the heart's contractions, in combination with an implantable cardiac defibrillator (ICD). Because Ambrose had left bundle branch block, he appeared to be an ideal candidate for CRT.

The therapy relies on a sophisticated battery-powered electronic pacing device (also called a biventricular pacemaker) that builds on technology used in traditional pacemakers. The CRT apparatus, which is surgically implanted under the skin, has three electrical wires positioned in the right atrium and right ventricle and into the *coronary sinus vein* to regulate the left ventricle. It fires small electrical impulses that the leads carry to the heart muscle, causing the left and right ventricles to contract and pump simultaneously, hence synchronizing the mechanical activity of the pumping chamber. CRT is always used in conjunction with medications for heart failure; the combination often brings about astounding improvement.

Within a day, Ambrose was approved for the CRT/ICD combination. Initially it appeared that we wouldn't be able to schedule the procedure until February. But this made Ambrose nervous. "I didn't want to go home," he says. "I was afraid. I thought, 'If I go home, I'm probably not coming back.'"

I agreed that the severity of Ambrose's heart failure and his bouts of fainting warranted juggling the schedule to book his surgery. Ambrose was moved up the list and received his biventricular ICD the next day, January 19.

The day after surgery, Ambrose visited the hospital's device clinic. Technicians there set the heart rate levels that would activate the device and check the function of the device and leads. With the biventricular ICD in place, Ambrose felt at ease for the first time in more than a month. "The doctors said it would keep my heart beating," he says. "That had always been my fear: that my heart was just going to quit. I felt more comfortable coming home."

Ambrose's CRT/ICD device also incorporated remote monitoring capabilities. Now I could check up on his condition by using a phone, computer, and system called CareLink that allows physicians to "interrogate" a pacemaker from anywhere in the world and see important information about the patient. We can determine his or her heart rhythm, heart rate, and activity level, as well as whether the person has been shocked for an arrhythmia. Some devices even allow doctors to see how much fluid may be accumulating in the lungs.

On the way back to Pennsylvania, Ambrose's thoughts once again turned to his sister. "She had a pacemaker, but that was it," he says. "Now four years later, medical advances had been made that gave me a better chance." Time would tell how much the medicines and CRT device could help his condition.

Following the doctor's orders

Doctors usually recommend that patients with heart failure continue medications throughout their lives. Even if a patient recovers and the ejection fraction normalizes, we believe that maintaining a stable condition is contingent upon taking proven medications, such as beta-blockers and ACE inhibitors. Doctors also believe that a CRT device is a lifelong form of therapy that has a good response. Ambrose will need to have new batteries implanted every three to five years and can also have the technology upgraded as advances occur.

Ambrose's condition has improved. A year and a half after the surgery, his ejection fraction was 40 percent, and his heart had shrunk to 5.7 centimeters, just slightly larger than a normal heart. Although the pacemaker component of his device is always working, the defibrillator has never gone off.

Another change in Ambrose is his weight: he is approximately 60 pounds lighter than prior to his diagnosis. The six-foot-three-inch man remains lean thanks to a low-fat, low-sodium diet. "I eat as much as I want, but I watch what I eat," he explains. Like all patients with heart failure, Ambrose was encouraged to limit his sodium and fluid intake. Today he still adheres diligently to that advice. "Every day, I write down what I eat, what I drink, and how much of it, so I know exactly how much sodium I have and how much fluid I drink," he says. He also takes his blood pressure, measures his pulse, and weighs himself each morning.

To some, that may seem a bit overboard, but Ambrose wants to enjoy life with his family and continue his favorite activities. He's back to golfing in the summer and walks and carries his bag when he plays nine holes. His only concession to his heart condition is that he'll ride in a golf cart if he plays 18.

Ambrose hunts again too. "I haven't pushed a real steep hill yet," he admits. "My kids won't let me do it! They tell me, 'Dad, you're not going where you used to.'" So he "only" climbs 80-foot hills as opposed to 100-foot ones.

Ambrose continues to work and is thankful that his employer is flexible about his schedule. He usually works in the morning, goes home for a 45-minute nap, then returns to the plant in the afternoon. "If I don't get my little nap in the middle of the day, my blood pressure drops, and I feel a little tired," he says.

Ambrose calls his biventricular ICD "a real lifesaver." The devices are new, so the long-term prognosis is unknown. But he's accepted the uncertainty and appreciates each day of good health. He sets aside time for fun and often takes spur-of-the-moment trips to visit his son in Washington, D.C.

"I put a little reminder sign up in my office," says Ambrose. "It reads, 'Take time, make the time, for there may not be another time.'"

Simple Ways to Monitor Heart Health at Home

Since undergoing cardiac resynchronization therapy in 2005, Ambrose has made regular follow-up visits to Cleveland Clinic. About once every three months, he has a checkup with me or another physician. But Ambrose keeps a close eye on his heart health at home, checking his pulse and monitoring his blood pressure daily.

Feeling your pulse to check your heart's rate, rhythm, and regularity is simple. Each pulse matches up with a heartbeat that pumps blood into the arteries. The force of the pulse helps calculate the amount of blood flow to the rest of your body. Your heart rate is the number of times your heart beats in one minute. At rest, a normal heart beats between 50 and 100 times per minute.

To measure your pulse, get a watch with a second hand. Place your index and middle fingers on the inner wrist of your other arm, just below the base of the thumb. You should feel a tapping or pulsing. Count the number of taps you feel in ten seconds, then multiply that number by 6 to determine your heart rate for one minute. When feeling your pulse, you also can tell whether your heart rhythm is regular or not. If you measure your pulse and blood pressure using one of the many home devices, there is a possibility that the readings may be inaccurate and not relate to how you feel. If you feel poorly, please consult with your physician.

Red Flag

Two simple clues to your heart—pulse and blood pressure—can reveal quite a bit about its health. If your resting heart rate is above 120 beats per minute or your typical blood pressure reading at rest or after activity changes significantly, contact your doctor.

Ambrose relies on a battery-operated gauge to monitor his blood pressure: the force that the blood exerts in the arteries as it's pumped throughout the body by the heart. Blood pressure records systolic pressure (pressure during the heart's contraction) and diastolic pressure (pressure when the heart relaxes between beats). For patients with heart failure, we usually advise that their blood pressure should be less than 120/80. If you don't have a blood pressure gauge at home, you can often find one at local pharmacies.

Chapter 11

A Long Journey to Success: Nancy's Story

"This past year, I've felt so good. I think it's the sum total of the biventricular pacemaker, my heart meds, and following the doctor's advice. I try not to let anything slow me down."

—Nancy, living with heart failure since being diagnosed at age 57 in 1991

During the summer of 2006, Nancy and her husband, Dick, took a leisurely cruise down the Mississippi River aboard a charming stern-wheeler. Along the way, they toured Civil War battlefields and antebellum homes, listened to soulful blues and jazz, and indulged in a little Cajun cuisine.

It was a memorable trip for the retired couple and amazing too, considering that 15 years earlier Nancy had received a dismal medical diagnosis. "Doctors told me I had cardiomyopathy and had only two to five years to live," she remembers.

Nancy has been my patient since 1992. During that time, I've treated hundreds of people with heart failure, but her story is one of the most remarkable. That's not because of her condition itself: Nancy has garden-variety dilated cardiomyopathy. Nor is it because she's received any revolutionary treatment, although she has certainly benefited from medical advances. Nancy is an inspiration because she's beaten the odds and leads a fulfilling life despite her heart failure.

I decided to end the patient-stories part of this book with Nancy's because she epitomizes the patients I mentioned in the introduction who have triumphed over their diagnoses. She's traveled the world and remains upbeat. People who want to hear an inspirational story of living a long, full life with heart failure should meet Nancy.

Nancy's Story: Respiratory Ailments and the Heart

While no one can say definitively what led to Nancy's cardiomyopathy, she suspects it was triggered in the late 1980s after she developed asthma and chronic sinus infections. "I've always been an outdoorsy person," says Nancy, whose beautiful flower garden, patio, and pond were once featured in her city's newspaper. "I'd rather work outside than inside."

In the fall of 1987, her mulching tractor broke, so Nancy raked the leaves in her acre-plus yard. "I inundated my lungs with leaf spores, and that brought my asthma to a head," she says. She also suffered a series of sinus infections. "My allergist and pulmonologist put me on high doses of prednisone to help me breathe."

Nancy's condition was so severe that she traveled all the way from Columbus, Ohio, to Denver's National Jewish Medical and Research Center, a leader in respiratory disorders. She participated in a weeklong class to learn how to manage her asthma better and reduce its side effects. Nancy was able to control her condition, but she believes that the combined effects of a compromised immune system and large doses of medication led to cardiomyopathy. "I think it lowered my resistance, and I picked up some virus," she speculates.

In 1991 Nancy began to experience the telltale shortness of breath that plagues so many patients with heart failure. "We have season tickets at the theater, and I could barely make it to our seats," she recalls. In addition, her feet and ankles began to swell.

"I told my allergist about the swelling, and he was quite alarmed," she says. "He put me in the hospital." Nancy spent 11 days there while physicians scrambled for answers. At one point, they thought she might have a gallbladder problem and considered removing the organ. However, before the surgery, a cardiologist was consulted.

"The cardiologist said, 'I think you have cardiomyopathy, but I don't know how to take care of it; I can't help you anymore,'" recalls Nancy. "In 1991 they just didn't know that much about it. I'm glad he was honest, but that was scary!" Lying in the hospital bed, surrounded by her family, Nancy realized that she needed a specialist.

"When I was released from the hospital," she says, "I looked around for another physician and found Dr. Starling."

Defying the prognosis

When I met Nancy, I was an assistant professor at the Ohio State University Hospitals in Columbus. I ordered numerous tests, including an electrocardiogram and an echocardiogram. Nancy's ejection fraction was only 10 percent. She also underwent cardiac catheterization to rule out blocked vessels or heart attack, and she had a heart biopsy, which indicated that her heart hadn't been weakened by active inflammation or myocarditis.

After determining that Nancy had dilated cardiomyopathy, probably caused by a virus, I placed her on an ACE inhibitor and a diuretic. I also suggested a low-sodium diet and exercise routine. With this course of treatment, I thought that Nancy had approximately two to five years to live.

"That scared me into making a big turnaround," says Nancy, who immediately reduced her salt intake—not a simple step in 1992. "If there were any low-sodium foods in the store, you had to climb up to the top shelves to find them. The food manufacturers are finally coming around."

Nancy also signed up for an exercise program for cardiac patients on the OSU campus. Three times a week, she rode a stationary bicycle or walked on a treadmill and performed conditioning exercises with elastic bands. She worked out alongside many heart failure patients waiting for heart transplants and nearly joined their ranks.

Exercise was not a standard recommendation 15 years ago; in fact, some cardiologists advised their patients against it. Today most specialists do recommend regular exercise for people with heart failure. (Exercise as a therapy for heart failure is currently the focus of a large clinical trial to provide definitive information. You can learn about the study—called HF-Action, for Heart Failure: A Controlled Trial Investigating Outcomes of Exercise TraiNing—online at *hfaction.org*.) But Nancy is a trailblazer, always seeking the newest and most promising treatment available.

Because of the gravity of her situation, I recommended that she undergo testing for a possible heart transplant. Nancy agreed and began the in-depth screening process. A team of cardiologists, nurses, social workers, and bioethicists began to review her medical history carefully, perform diagnostic tests and psychological evaluations, and compile her social history. The ultimate goal was to decide whether Nancy was a good candidate not only to survive the procedure but to comply with the need for continuous care afterward.

"It takes awhile to do all the testing," says Nancy. "With the regimen Dr. Starling gave me—the low-sodium diet, exercises, and heart medication—I started getting better. When it came time to put me on the transplant list, I said, 'I'm feeling good enough that I don't think I really have to do this.'" So Nancy held off going active on the transplant list. And she held on to her lifestyle for a dozen years.

Nancy continued working as the business manager at her husband's orthodontics practice, a job she'd held most of her married life. She faithfully exercised and took her ACE inhibitor and diuretic, plus a beta-blocker I'd added to her list of medications in 2000. "It's a pain to take a handful of medicine each morning and evening, but you can't forget," she emphasizes.

Otherwise, says Nancy, "I didn't really let the heart failure change my life." She buzzed around town in her beloved black Porsche. Nancy and Dick traveled frequently, their trips including a vacation to the Greek islands and five cruises. Once a year, Nancy had checkups with me at Cleveland Clinic, where I was appointed to the cardiovascular medicine department in 1995. In between, she checked in with her cardiologist in Columbus.

An extraordinary turnaround

Through the years, Nancy's ejection fraction has hovered between 10 percent and 20 percent. "It's always been so low that when physicians look at me, they can't understand how I walk around and do so much," she says. Nancy also developed a bundle branch block that prevented her left and right ventricles from contracting simultaneously.

During a checkup in November 2004, I suggested that she receive a biventricular pacemaker and defibrillator. The implantable device would help the ventricles pump in sync, as well as shock Nancy's heart back into rhythm if necessary.

"At the time Dr. Starling recommended the device, I felt good," says Nancy. "I asked him why I should do this. He said it would help me out now and in the future. Then he said, 'If you were my mother, I'd tell you to do this.' So I said okay."

Nancy received her biventricular pacer and defibrillator in January 2005. She spent two nights at the clinic; her biggest complaint being muscle soreness where the pacemaker leads had been threaded. "It does hurt, but it's something you grin and bear because it's ultimately going to be helpful," she says.

In the fall of 2006, Nancy came to me for another checkup. While we chatted, she mentioned that after living with heart failure for 15 years, she doubted that her condition was going to get better. I agreed that most people's hearts don't improve dramatically after being weakened and enlarged for so many years. Later I received the results of her echocardiogram, and they proved me wrong!

Nancy's ejection fraction was whopping 55 percent. I couldn't believe it. I called the head of the echo lab and asked whether her echocardiograms could have been misread. But the number was accurate. I was so excited that I called Nancy with the good news from my mobile phone on the drive home that night.

In the years since, Nancy's heart has shrunk and her EF has risen even further. "I really feel good," she says. Nancy continues to take her medication, watch her diet, and walk on her treadmill 35 minutes a day, except for Sundays. "The most important thing is to do exactly what your doctor tells you to do," she advises other heart failure patients.

That's deceptively simple advice. And there is no simple answer for why Nancy's heart has recovered. But some of it must be attributed to her strong spirit. "I don't really let things bother me," she says. "I know what has to be done, I know my limitations, and I go from there."

And Nancy and Dick certainly are on the go. This year they're planning a trip to Arizona to visit friends and another to a convention in Pennsylvania for people who collect ice cream memorabilia. "There's no sense going in reverse," Nancy reflects. "You won't be very happy. You have to be the captain of your own ship."

Nancy returned for her annual checkup in August 2007, telling me that she feels the best she has in more than ten years. Nancy and I held our breath before her annual echo was completed, and ultimately the news was good: her heart was pumping normally, and its size was normal, thanks to medication, a biventricular pacemaker, and Nancy's dedication to her self-care.

New Options on the Horizon

As of March 2007, the U.S. National Institutes of Health listed more than 360 federally and privately supported clinical trials for heart failure on its Web site, ClinicalTrials.gov. At renowned institutions and hospitals across the nation, researchers are aggressively working to enhance patients' lifestyles through new medications, surgical treatments, and assist devices. They're also studying prevention, diagnostic,

Researching Clinical Trials

ClinicalTrials.gov provides details about each trial's purpose, eligibility criteria, and phone numbers for more information. Information there should be used in conjunction with advice from health care professionals. To begin your online search, you may want to start on the resources page (*clinicaltrials.gov/ct2/info/resources*), which provides general information about clinical trials. You also can use the Web site's search engine, typing in "heart failure," to find specific trials on the condition.

early intervention, caregiving, and end-stage heart failure options.

It would require a book of its own to describe all the cutting-edge research and clinical trials currently being conducted. Most heart failure centers offer evidence-based therapies in addition to new and evolving therapies being studied in clinical trials. Here is just a sampling of some of the basic research, heart failure therapy studies, and cardio-vascular surgery research that's being carried out at just one institution: the George M. and Linda H. Kaufman Center for Heart Failure at Cleveland Clinic.

- Surgeons at the Kaufman Center and researchers in the clinic's Lerner Research Center are developing innovative blood pump technology, including the PediPump, an implantable pediatric ventricular assist device, and a new and smaller total artificial heart.

- The department of cardiovascular medicine conducts electrophysiology studies to determine the subcellular basis for atrial fibrillation and the increased arrhythmias associated with heart failure.

- The Kaufman Center has commenced clinical trials utilizing a left ventricular assist device as permanent treatment for end-stage heart failure patients who are not candidates for heart transplants. The use of mechanical devices is growing, and technology and outcomes are improving.

- Physicians are involved in a multicenter international study for patients with coronary heart disease and heart failure, investigating surgical treatment for ischemic heart failure, including the latest advances with stem cell treatments.

- Physicians are studying patients with acute and chronic cardiomyopathy, hoping to identify and treat these ailments better by understanding the genetics and triggers for cardiomyopathy.

- There is ongoing research into new medications and devices.

Cardiac transplantation remains the most effective treatment for patients who have progressed to end-stage heart failure. But physicians and researchers alike remain optimistic that the considerable pharmacological and surgical advances being made each day can slow the disease's progression and extend patients' lives. Cardiologists like me know that heart transplantation can save lives, but we continue our efforts to improve treatments and reverse—even prevent—heart disease. Our goal is for patients to live long and productive lives with their own hearts.

PART III

Conclusion

Chapter 12

Living with Heart Failure

R oughly 15 years ago, a patient would have been given medication, then asked to wait for a heart transplant while his or her condition deteriorated. Today there are many more medical options, and more patients with heart failure are living longer. Medical advances, new devices, and treatments have been important. Finding the cause of heart failure, when possible, is essential. Also essential: patients must share actively in the recovery process and follow doctors' guidelines.

Frank

At age 55, Frank was still the life of the party. He and his wife would clear out their living room furniture, set up blackjack and craps tables, and invite friends to casino parties. Each August they traveled to South Carolina's Hilton Head Island, where Frank played a little tennis and ate a lot of spicy buffalo wings, which he washed down with beer.

As a marketing executive for sports talk radio stations, Frank even held a job that was equal parts festivity and work. He sold advertising space to beer companies and lined up sponsorships for sports-related events, such as the Corona Buckeye Bash held at a restaurant in Columbus, Ohio, when the Ohio State football team faced the University of Texas Longhorns. "You go there to work, but you party a little," admits Frank. "You certainly want to sample your clients' products!"

But years of this lifestyle took their toll on the middle-aged man. All his life, Frank had been an athlete, playing football and basketball in school, then joining bowling, racquetball, and basketball leagues as an adult. Despite being physically active, Frank didn't watch his diet and gained weight. Then in the summer of 2005, he began experiencing shortness of breath.

Frank felt pressure in his chest, and his legs ached while mowing the lawn. Walking through the airport on his annual trip to Hilton Head, he stopped to rest a few times. Then while playing tennis with his son, Frank was unable to catch his breath and spent the night coughing on the couch.

In September Frank visited his doctor, who sent him to the hospital for tests. His blood pressure was high, his heart rate was 145 beats per minute, and his ejection fraction was 10 percent. Frank was diagnosed with cardiomyopathy. He came to Cleveland Clinic for help in October.

I realized that Frank didn't take very good care of himself and encouraged him to stop drinking and eat a healthy diet. In addition, I prescribed a beta-blocker, a cholesterol-lowering medication, a diuretic, and an ARB vasodilator to get his heart back in rhythm and improve his condition.

I also recognized immediately that Frank's rapid heart rate, an arrhythmia, could be the cause of his cardiomyopathy. That was actually good news, because it meant that we might have a chance to reverse the disease and get him back to normal. However, Frank was quite ill, so I decided to admit him to the hospital upon his first visit to get him "tuned up" and to remove fluids from his body.

After an echocardiogram looking for blood clots, we started Frank on a antiarrhythmia medication called amiodarone. We were able to slow down his heart rate, and eventually his heart returned to a regular rhythm. Then we decided to wait and hope that the combination of medications, a regular heart rhythm, and a healthy lifestyle—including absolutely no alcohol—would correct the heart problem.

Frank did begin feeling better but was still sluggish. His ejection fraction rose to nearly 40 percent. Yet he still was at risk to have recurrent arrhythmias, so Frank underwent a catheter ablation in February 2006. In this procedure, a catheter is inserted into the heart, and a special machine delivers energy precisely to miniscule areas of the heart muscle that are causing abnormal rhythms. The goal is for the electrical impulses to disconnect the pathway of the abnormal rhythm. The ablation was *successful, and Frank's heart has remained in normal rhythm ever since.*

Today, thanks to the procedure, medication, and lifestyle changes, Frank is healthier and feels terrific. His heart size has decreased, and his EF is 55 percent. He no longer takes a blood thinner or amiodarone, although he will continue the beta-blocker and ARB indefinitely. Frank eats a low-sodium diet, works out regularly on an elliptical machine, watches his fluid intake, and has stopped drinking alcohol. He has lost more than 50 pounds since his first visit to see me. None of the changes has been easy, he says, but you need to "work with your doctors and keep your chin up."

Many of the suggestions made to people with heart failure are beneficial to anyone's health, such as better eating habits and a regular exercise program. This chapter covers several ways that you can improve your chances for a longer, happier life, while managing your heart failure.

Stay in Touch with Your Health Care Team

Even if you think you have your condition under control, it's important to maintain regular follow-up appointments with your doctor. Sustaining a relationship with health care providers helps increase the likelihood that you'll remain on your treatment path and stay healthy.

You may visit your doctor only a few times per year, so keep track of your condition in between visits. Nancy, my 73-year-old patient who has lived with heart failure for 16 years, keeps a medical log. Because she suffers from asthma and sinus infections in addition to heart failure, Nancy meticulously tracks the medications she takes and any procedures she undergoes. She also records doctor visits, logging the name of the physician, his or her phone number, and the reason for the appointment. This way, she explains, "when I go to a different physician, he can get a rough idea of what I've been through."

Talk to your doctor about getting an annual flu shot and a pneumonia vaccine every five years to avoid illness, and check with your doctor before you take any over-the-counter medications. Also mention any big plans or events that might add stress to your life or require special medical care, such as vacations or weddings. A year and a half after my patient Jennifer received a heart transplant, she planned a trip to Jamaica. Prior to leaving, she got a hepatitis A shot.

Remember Your Medication

For nine years, 48-year-old MaryBeth has taken a beta-blocker and ACE inhibitor to treat her heart failure. Over time, some patients begin to skip dosages, but not MaryBeth. "I do not forget my medicine," she says. "If it's a matter of taking three pills a day, I certainly don't mind. It's a small price to pay."

For more and more heart failure patients, a combination of medications is the key to managing their condition—or even reversing the symptoms, in some cases. But it's critical for patients to know the names, dosages, and side effects of all their prescriptions. You must fill your prescriptions regularly and take them as scheduled, at the same time each day, and precisely as prescribed.

Watch Your Weight

It's important for heart failure patients to hop on a scale each day, for weight is one indicator of heart function. Changes may point to fluid retention or signal that your condition is worsening or your medication isn't working. Here are a few tips for your daily weigh-in:

- Use the same scale and wear similar clothing for consistency.
- Weigh yourself at the same time each day. Do it after urinating and prior to eating.
- Keep track of your weight in a diary or on a calendar.
- Check for increased swelling, which indicates fluid retention. You may be retaining fluid if your belt feels tighter, your stomach seems swollen, your clothes are snug, or your shoes seem tight. If so, eliminate 500 milligrams of sodium and decrease liquids by 1½ cups for two days; if you don't notice a decrease in body fluid or weight afterward, call your doctor.

- Call your physician or nurse if you gain three or more pounds in one day or five or more pounds in a week.

Monitor Your Fluids

It is likely that your doctor will restrict the amount you drink each day. While fluid intake varies by patient, a common recommendation is approximately 2 liters (equal to 8¼ cups or 66 ounces) every 24 hours.

It's a good idea to write down what you drink to help ensure that you're not taking in too many fluids. Don't forget to track fluid foods too, such as soup and ice cream. One method that helps some patients get a handle on fluid intake is to fill a two-quart pitcher or two-liter soda bottle to the top. Place the filled container in your kitchen. Each time you drink or eat something fluid, pour out the same amount of liquid from the container. When it's empty, you've reached your daily limit.

In time, restricting your fluids will become a habit, and you may not need to track them so diligently. You may also record your urine output to make sure that you're not ingesting too many liquids. Another note: if you're thirsty, don't assume that your body needs more fluids. By drinking too much, you'll offset the benefits of your diuretic. You can alleviate thirst by sucking on ice chips or hard candy or chewing sugarless gum. Covering your lips with lip balm may help too.

Follow a Healthy Diet

When MaryBeth shops for her family, she typically selects fresh fruit and vegetables and avoids canned goods and other processed food. The family has also eliminated salt from its diet. While the shift in eating habits took some getting used to, it's now second nature. "We've adapted, and I don't feel like it's a big change anymore," says MaryBeth.

One of the most important steps in managing heart failure is to control sodium intake. Salt contributes to water retention, which can lead to swelling. Your doctor can tell you how much sodium you may consume daily, but general guidelines from the Heart Failure Society of America recommend between 2,000 and 3,000 milligrams, depending on the severity of your condition. To put this in perspective, a teaspoon of table salt contains 2,300 milligrams of sodium. It takes effort to reduce sodium intake.

It helps to practice good nutritional habits in general, as MaryBeth does. Fresh vegetables and fruits, lean meats, dried beans, and whole-grain bread are all healthy choices that are naturally low in sodium. If you opt for canned goods and other processed food, choose ones labeled "sodium free" or "low sodium" and check the nutritional information.

To offset the fatigue common in heart failure patients, consider adding foods rich in potassium to your diet. These include bananas, strawberries, citrus fruit, spinach, broccoli, and carrots. Also choose foods high in fiber, such as whole grains, bran, fruits, and vegetables. Decreasing calories and achieving your ideal body weight will help you manage your condition too. Bear in mind that if you are anticoagulated, certain types of vegetables, typically greens, can affect your coagulation blood test.

Exercise Regularly

Some types of physical activity may be off-limits. For instance, before my patient Joe had his heart attack and was subsequently diagnosed with heart failure, he used to swim in the ocean at his summer home in New Jersey. But because swimming requires constantly lifting his arms over his head, he can no longer do it. Now he walks several miles each day.

It's important for people with heart failure to get plenty of rest to prevent exhaustion. That may include a short nap during the day. However, it's equally important to stay active. If you don't exercise, your muscles won't produce as much energy. And as your energy wanes, your heart needs to pump more blood to your muscles. That increased pumping stresses the heart.

Regular aerobic exercise, such as walking or biking, strengthens the heart. It improves the muscles' efficiency in using oxygen and increases blood flow to arms and legs. Check with your physician before you pursue an exercise regimen, then plan a set time each day to work out. You might select the morning, when your energy is at its peak. You may also consider starting out slowly: park your car farther from stores so that you walk some more or take a couple flights of stairs rather than use the elevator.

Soon you will see the positive results of regular exercise. Since June 2005, my patient Ambrose has walked three miles daily. "I'm probably in better shape now than I was before," he says. Nancy, who is now 73, exercises every day! We know that exercise is beneficial for everyone, even patients with heart failure. But common sense is always the best guide. More scientific information will soon be available when the results of a large prospective trial (mentioned in chapter 10) studying the benefits of exercise in heart failure patients is completed. For now, ask your doctor for guidelines.

Manage Your Symptoms

In all the patient case studies in this book, one recurrent symptom appeared: shortness of breath. Although it's arguably the most common complaint of heart failure patients, there are ways to improve your breathing. Try interspersing periods of activity with times of rest. Relax in a chair with your feet up and listen to music, watch a favorite TV show, meditate, or read.

Avoid extreme temperatures, as very hot or cold weather may exacerbate your symptoms. High humidity, in particular, can cause fatigue. Over time, you'll learn how to manage your condition. When Nancy took a summer cruise down the Mississippi River, she realized that it would be a muggy trip. She still enjoyed the daily excursions when the ship docked, but she didn't climb hills, and she wore a large, floppy hat to avoid direct sunlight and stay cooler.

If breathlessness persists at night, you may prop yourself up with more pillows or sleep in a recliner. Also, stay away from strenuous household chores such as heavy lifting, shoveling snow, or scrubbing floors. In addition, protect your overall health by staying clear of people who have colds, bronchitis, the flu, or other infectious diseases.

More importantly, a change in your symptoms could signal the need to change medications or that something else requires attention. Please call your doctor promptly to discuss any new symptoms.

Many people with heart failure resume normal routines and return to work. You may start back to work gradually. You may, however, need to shift your career focus if your job requires physical exertion. Prior to Dan's diagnosis with heart failure, he was a tree cutter. When his condition worsened, he went to college and began working as a researcher on natural resources for a university. When Dan fell gravely ill and required a heart transplant, he stopped work completely. Seven months after his transplant, Dan returned to the job part time. For three months, he worked 20 hours a week. In May 2006, he resumed work full time. "I feel great," he says.

Above all, ask for help from family and friends if you need it and don't be too proud to rely on assist devices, such as walkers and shower chairs, if necessary.

Cope with Your Feelings

After MaryBeth received an implantable defibrillator in 1999, I suggested that she join a 12-week cardiac rehabilitation program at her local hospital. The attendees met three times a week for exercise and classes on managing their heart conditions. While the class itself was valuable, perhaps the greatest benefit for MaryBeth was bonding with other patients. In particular, she looked forward to talking to a man about her age who'd had a heart attack. "The program gave me a lot of confidence that I'd be okay," says MaryBeth.

Joining a support group can be quite helpful. It's not uncommon for people living with ongoing conditions such as heart failure to become worried or depressed. As you take control of your health and follow the guidelines in this chapter, such feelings are likely to fade. But it helps to chat with others in the same boat. If you're uncomfortable attending a support group, then consider one-on-one counseling with a trained therapist or spiritual leader.

There are other ways to keep the blues at bay. Make sure you get dressed and out of the house everyday, even if it's only for a short walk. Try to maintain the hobbies that interested you previously, though you may have to modify them upon your doctor's recommendations. For instance, if you were an avid golfer, limit yourself to 9 holes rather than 18 and use a golf cart instead of walking. Get a good night's sleep and set realistic goals for what you can accomplish each day.

Some Parting Thoughts

In this book, you have met ten of my patients, all of whom are living with heart failure. Not everyone diagnosed with the condition will meet with the same success as Dan, Mike,

Nancy, and the others, but medical advancements continue rapidly and more people are leading satisfying lives.

I have been a cardiac physician for 20 years and have treated countless heart failure patients. My motivation for writing this book is to share with you the common themes and experiences of patients, even though they have different forms of heart failure.

It was important to them, and will be to you, to find the right person to help guide you through your journey. As you have read, cardiologists now have many new developments in their toolkits to treat heart failure. Many new ones are being developed as our understanding improves.

It is important that you have confidence in the person and the health care institution that will guide you through your journey, no matter what the final destination. Your confidence will be more secure if your provider has the right level of expertise and can utilize all the evidence-based treatments available.

I will leave the final words to Stephen, whose letter prefaces this book:

I hope in reading this book you have come to see that the future can be promising. Your choice of doctor and institution is instrumental in making sure that future is a promising as possible. In my travels, I have been cared for by a great many doctors, most of whom have been fabulous. Those I trust the most have three things in common. They have many years of focused experience and have treated thousands of patients; they have seen it all. Secondly, they work for the finest institutions, recognized for their leadership in health care, not just in cardiology. Finally, and possibly most importantly, I have confidence that even if the test results indicate I am fine, they will relentlessly continue their investigations, searching for why I feel under the weather.

So work with your doctor, be an advocate for your own health, and be optimistic for the future. You will find you are on a journey of hope, challenge, and success.

Acknowledgments

I thank my many patients and my family for making this book possible. My wife has supported me throughout my career, and this book would never have happened without her enduring support. I sincerely thank Carl V. Leier, MD, for starting me on this journey and being my mentor.

Appendix 1

Comfort Care for a Chronic Illness

Even with advances in medical technology and improved prognoses for many heart failure patients, the condition is often fatal. While extending the lifespan of most patients is a laudable goal, it's also important to focus attention on palliative care—to make sure that people with heart failure are as comfortable as possible at the end of their lives when treatments prove unsuccessful.

Top-notch palliative care can help ease a person's suffering. As a patient or a family member of someone with heart failure, you should openly discuss end-of-life issues with doctors and nurses. Chronic illnesses are stressful for everyone involved. Planning for the future while patients are still relatively healthy helps everyone make the best possible choices and prepare for eventual death.

It's often difficult to forecast the length of survival in heart failure patients; many live years longer than physicians originally predicted. But for patients in the end stages of heart failure, the emphasis should be on keeping them comfortable; relieving pain and symptoms, such as labored breathing; and maintaining as much function for as long as possible.

The following are some considerations for palliative care:

Inotropic therapy. Designed to stimulate a weak heart to work harder, inotropic drugs administered intravenously are used in end-stage heart failure to help alleviate and control symptoms so you can better perform your daily activities. Such inotropic therapies are used only when oral medication no longer works. Common inotropics include dobutamine and milrinone.

Home health care services. Registered nurses who offer home care can be an asset to heart failure patients and their families. They provide a range of services and advice, from how to care for intravenous sites, catheters, and infusion pumps to how to handle dying at home.

Spiritual and emotional well-being. Equally important to physical comfort is ensuring that you and your family have come to terms with the process of dying. Communicate your preferences and hopes for an easy death: When do you want to turn off your ICD defibrillator if it's firing frequently? Do you want to die at home if possible? Do you have an updated living will or durable power of attorney and a do-not-resuscitate (DNR) order? Consider talking to your priest, minister, rabbi, or another spiritual advisor about end-of-life issues.

Patient control. Patients should be given as much autonomy as possible. They should have choices related to diet, fluids, and their medical plan.

Appendix 2

Online Resources

American Heart Association
americanheart.org

Cardiomyopathy Association
cardiomyopathy.org

CHFpatients.com
chfpatients.com

Cleveland Clinic Kaufman Center for Heart Failure
my.clevelandclinic.org/heart/heartfailure

ClinicalTrials.gov
clinicaltrials.gov

Heart Failure Society of America
hfsa.org

HeartHealthyWomen.org
hearthealthywomen.org

Heartmates (for caregivers)
heartmates.com

International Society for Heart & Lung Transplantation
ishlt.org

*i*Village YourTotalHealth's Heart Health Center
yourtotalhealth.ivillage.com/heart-health

The Mended Hearts (for caregivers)
mendedhearts.org

National Caregivers Library
caregiverslibrary.org

National Coalition for Women with Heart Disease
womenheart.org

National Family Caregivers Association
nfcacares.org

National Heart, Lung, and Blood Institute
www.nhlbi.nih.gov

National Women's Health Information Center
4women.gov

OrganDonor.Gov
organdonor.gov

Organ Procurement and Transplantation Network
www.optn.org

United Network for Organ Sharing
unos.org

*Web*MD's **theheart.org**
theheart.org

Well Spouse Association *(for caregivers)*
wellspouse.org

Glossary

Anemia (also anaemia): lack of oxygen in the blood

Aneurysm: when part of an artery becomes enlarged and expands making the vessel wall weak

Aorta: a large artery which carries oxygenated blood from the heart to the rest of the body

Aortic valve: the valve in the heart which controls the flow of blood from the heart into the aorta

Arrhythmia: an irregular heartbeat

Artery: a blood vessel that carries blood away from the heart

Atria (also Atriums): collectively both upper chambers of the heart

Biventricular: relating to both right and left ventricles

Blood chemistry: all the testable chemicals contained in the blood

Cardiomyopathy: a disease of the heart muscle

Cardiotoxic: doing damage to the heart

Catheter: a tube, lead or wire that is inserted into the body through an appropriate channel

Catheterization: the process of inserting a catheter

Chemotherapy: the use of certain types of drugs to destroy cancerous cells

Chromosomes: a collection of 22 DNA bundles that provide the genetic code for life

Contrast: a special chemical which helps improve medical imaging results

Diastolic: related to the period during which the heart relaxes and expands

Defibrillator: an implanted device which monitors the heart rhythm and can shock and pace the heart back to normal rhythm if is going dangerously fast

Digoxin: a drug used to treat certain heart conditions including heart failure and atrial arrhythmias

Diuretic: drug that encourages urination

Doppler Effect: the change in the detectable wave frequency due to their direction of travel

Doppler echocardiogram: a special type of echocardiogram that images blood flows by measuring the Doppler Effect in the movement of blood

Echocardiogram (Echo): a way of imaging the moving heart using sound waves

Edema (also Oedema): an abnormal accumulation of fluid in the body tissue

Electrode: small patches with gentle adhesive that when applied to the skin allow the electrical activity of the body to be measured

Electrolytes: chemicals that are capable of conducting electrical energy measured in the blood

Electrophysiology: the study of the electrical properties and activity of cells, most commonly in the heart

Embolism: the result of an abnormal movement of a substance that results in a blockage, often in a blood vessel

Endocarditis: an infection of the inner lining of the heart and valves

Hematoma: an area of internal bleeding forming a clot

Hypertension: a condition in which the blood pressure is abnormally high

Hypotension: a condition in which the blood pressure is abnormally low

Intravenous: administering medication directly into a vein

Ischemia: the restriction of blood flow due to a blockage impairing heart muscle function

Lipid disorder: problems in the production of cholesterol and triglycerides

Myocardium: the muscle from which the heart is composed

Pacemaker: an implanted device that helps maintain the appropriate heart rhythm

Peripartum: on or around the time of childbirth

Plaque: fats within or attached to the walls of arteries which can restrict blood flow

Positron: atomic particles which carry a positive charge and are the opposite of electrons

Pulmonologist: a doctor specializing in diseases of the lung

Rheumatic fever: an inflammatory disease which affects several parts of the body, including the heart

Septal: of, or relating to the septum

Septum: the wall that divides two areas or chambers, in this instance the chambers of the heart

Stethoscope: a device which allows a doctor to listen to the internal noises of a body

Subcellular: existing or located within a cell

Thyroid: a gland in the neck which regulates a number of important chemical processes in the body

Topical anesthetic: a localized anesthetic used on the surface of skin or tissue

Transesophageal: quite literally to cross (pass through) the esophagus (throat)

Vein: a blood vessel that carries blood towards the heart

Ventricles: the two large (and lower) chambers of the heart

Virus: an agent which can only reproduce within a host cell

X-ray: a form of electromagnetic radiation which can generate images of certain parts within the body.

Index

About the Author

Randall C. Starling, MD, MPH, is Head of the Section of Heart Failure and Cardiac Transplant Medicine, the Medical Director of the Kaufman Center for Heart Failure, and a Staff Cardiologist in the Cleveland Clinic Department of Cardiovascular Medicine. He also serves as Vice Chairman of Cardiovascular Medicine, Operations. He is Professor of Medicine at the Cleveland Clinic Lerner College of Medicine, Case Western Reserve Univeristy.

Dr. Starling specializes in congestive heart failure, cardiac transplantation, cardiomyopathy, and mechanical circulatory support devices. Dr. Starling was appointed to the Cleveland Clinic in 1995. He is a Fellow in the American College of Cardiology and a member of the American Heart Association Council on Clinical Cardiology, the American Society of Transplantation, the Heart Failure Society of America, and the International Society for Heart and Lung Transplantation. He serves on the board of directors of the International Society of Heart and Lung Transplantation and the Executive Council for the Heart Failure Society of America.

Dr. Starling is a native of Pittsburgh, Pennsylvania, and attended the University of Pittsburgh, earning a BS in biology and an MD from Temple University in Philadelphia, Pennsylvania Dr. Starling earned a Masters in Public Health from the University of Pittsburgh Graduate School of Public Health. He has been an active researcher throughout his career and has authored more than 300 articles, abstracts, and book chapters. Dr Starling enjoys teaching and regularly educates medical students, nurses, residents, fellows, and physicians.

About Stephen Bacon

Stephen Bacon is a patient at Cleveland Clinic. He had his first pacemaker at 19 years of age, having inherited cardiomyopathy from his mother. After developing heart failure in 2003, he sold the company he had founded and run for 17 years, making a new career for himself as an independent business consultant. He is currently listed for a heart transplant, and is writing a book about his experiences as a heart patient. In his spare time he cooks, seeking to prove that low sodium food can be tasty. Stephen lives in Cambridge, England.

About Cleveland Clinic

Cleveland Clinic, located in Cleveland, Ohio, is a not-for-profit multispecialty academic medical center that integrates clinical and hospital care with research and education.

Cleveland Clinic was founded in 1921 by four renowned physicians with a vision of providing outstanding patient care based upon the principles of cooperation, compassion and innovation. *U.S. News & World Report* consistently names Cleveland Clinic as one of the nation's best hospitals in its annual "America's Best Hospitals" survey.

Approximately 1,800 full-time salaried physicians and researchers at Cleveland Clinic and Cleveland Clinic Florida represent more than 100 medical specialties and subspecialties. In 2007, there were 3.5 million outpatient visits to Cleveland Clinic and 50,455 hospital admissions. Patients came for treatment from every state and from more than 80 countries. Cleveland Clinic's Web site address is *clevelandclinic.org.*